Transient Global Amnesia

A.J. Larner

Transient Global Amnesia

From Patient Encounter to Clinical
Neuroscicncc

Second Edition

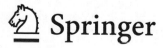 Springer

A.J. Larner
Cognitive Function Clinic
Walton Centre for Neurology and Neurosurgery
Liverpool, UK

ISBN 978-3-030-98941-5   ISBN 978-3-030-98939-2   (eBook)
https://doi.org/10.1007/978-3-030-98939-2

This Springer imprint is published by the registered company Springer Nature Switzerland AG
The registered company address is: Gewerbestrasse 11, 6330 Cham, Switzerland

Foreword to the Second Edition

Transient global amnesia (TGA) is amongst the most dramatic and distinctive cognitive disorders—the abrupt loss of the ability to lay down any conscious memory of continuing events, combined with a more variable loss of recall for recent events, bewilders sufferers and alarms their companions in equal measure. Mercifully, rather than being the harbinger of disaster that it at first appears, the condition is typically benign. It offers a striking glimpse of brain mechanisms—revealing that abilities we normally take to be integral to our human minds are in fact dissociable, as patients with TGA suddenly enter, and then just as mysteriously depart, the deeply disconcerting predicament of amnesia. The condition defies the false dichotomy between neurology and psychiatry—emotional stress is a recognised trigger of this thoroughly 'neurological' condition. And it is important clinically—sufficiently common that every casualty officer should be able to identify and manage it, not least to avoid the risk of prescribing powerful but unnecessary treatment for a suspected stroke.

Whilst it is distinctive, revealing, common, and clinically important, its pathophysiology remains a major puzzle. Successive attempts to explain TGA as a kind of epilepsy, a form of vascular event, and a variety of migraine have failed, although each of these disorders shares a fascinating border zone with TGA. Transient epileptic amnesia, transient ischaemic amnesia, transient migrainous amnesia, and TGA, all discussed in this volume, give to recognisably different, if sometimes overlapping, presentations. Nevertheless, occasional patients still defy our best efforts at classification. As Andrew discusses, TGA may in fact reflect a unique form of pathology, in keeping with the unique contribution of the medial temporal lobes to memory processing.

So memorable to clinicians is TGA at first encounter that it has been an exceptionally fertile source of case reports. Whilst these singular encounters are the place where medical science takes off, making systematic sense of TGA has required the creation of registries of carefully studied cases, epidemiological analyses, and, increasingly, the application of modern imaging techniques linked to contemporary models of memory systems and processes. Andrew outlines what we have learned from each of these sources.

v

The subject of TGA has been much in need of a thoughtful synthesis which Andrew supplies in this enlightening monograph. In the current academic world, scientists—in my view—write too many papers but too few books. Books allow their authors space to place subjects in their historical context, pull together the strands of evidence, bring order to a mass of disparate clues. We owe Andrew a debt for taking the time to write *Transient Global Amnesia*, and for his scholarly and rigorous treatment of this intriguing disorder. This volume will be the first place young clinicians and researchers intrigued by TGA should look to inform themselves fully—and an equally valuable resource for the seasoned operator.

Adam Zeman
Professor of Cognitive and Behavioural Neurology
University of Exeter College of Medicine and Health
St Luke's Campus
Exeter, UK

Preface to the First Edition [2017]

This book has evolved from more than 15 years of personal experience in seeing patients with transient global amnesia (TGA) as one component of work in a dedicated cognitive disorders clinic based at a regional neurosciences centre (Larner 2014), as well as in general neurology clinics and on ward consultation visits in district and teaching hospitals served by the centre and to which I have been assigned. However, my interest in TGA dates back around 30 years to medical student days in Oxford (1984–7) which happened to coincide with the time that John Hodges' studies of the condition were in progress. Twenty-five years on, his monograph (Hodges 1991) remains a seminal work in the field, even though it predates the explosion of neuroimaging studies using various modalities which were unavailable at that time. The only other book-length treatments of TGA are, to my knowledge (largely confined as it is to the English language), those of Markowitsch (1990) and, most recently, Britt Talley Daniel (2012).

Nevertheless, despite the paucity of books, many reviews have been (e.g. Whitty 1977, Caplan 1985; Kritchevsky 1992; Zeman and Hodges 1997) and continue to be published on the subject (e.g. considering only the past 10 years or so, Sander and Sander 2005; Butler and Zeman 2006; Quinette et al. 2006; Simos and Papanicolaou 2006; Owen et al. 2007; Marin-Garcia and Ruiz-Vargas 2008; Shekhar 2008; Veran et al. 2008; Klötzsch 2009; Bartsch and Deuschl 2010; Urban 2010; Hunter 2011; Kirshner 2011; Forman 2012; Bartsch and Butler 2013; Marazzi et al. 2014; Szabo 2014; Wilkinson and Derry 2014; Arena and Rabinstein 2015), including brief accounts from this centre (Larner 2008a, b, 2013; Larner et al. 2011; Williamson and Larner 2015). These publications attest to the interest in the condition of not only neurologists but also general physicians, emergency room specialists (Brown 1997; Harrison and Williams 2007; Faust and Nemes 2016), psychiatrists, occupational health physicians, and even practitioners involved in medico-legal work (Griebe et al. 2015), all of whom may encounter TGA patients. Moreover, amongst neurologists, not only those with an interest in cognitive neurology but also specialists in headache disorders, epilepsy, and stroke may need to consider TGA in the differential diagnosis of their typical patient cohorts. Hence a broad constituency of clinicians may require access to a ready source of information about TGA, presenting a lacuna for a further synoptic account of the condition. This is supplemented by my own clinical experience, with illustrative case material summarised in occasional Case Study text boxes.

This is a book by a clinician for clinicians which also delves a little into the brain-behaviour implications (the neuropsychology of mental structure) of the condition, hence the arrangement of the chapters: after a brief overview of the historical perspective (Chap. 1), the clinical aspects are covered (Chaps. 2–5) before a review of epidemiology and aetiopathogenesis (Chaps. 6 and 7, respectively). The book does not aim to review, far less to catalogue, every paper ever written on the subject of TGA, and in view of previous extensive reviews (e.g. Quinette et al. 2006) the focus is particularly on material published in the past 10 years. Although the book builds on the work of many clinicians, any remaining errors and misconceptions are my own.

Liverpool, UK   A.J. Larner

References

Arena JE, Rabinstein AA. Transient global amnesia. Mayo Clin Proc. 2015;90:264–72.

Bartsch T, Butler C. Transient amnesic syndromes. Nat Rev Neurol. 2013;9:86–97.

Bartsch T, Deuschl G. Transient global amnesia: functional anatomy and clinical implications. Lancet Neurol. 2010;9:205–14.

Brown J. ED evaluation of transient global amnesia. Ann Emerg Med. 1997;30:522–6.

Butler C, Zeman A. Syndromes of transient amnesia. Adv Clin Neurosci Rehabil. 2006;6(4):13–4.

Caplan LB [sic]. Transient global amnesia. In: Frederiks JAM, editor. Handbook of clinical neurology. Volume 1 (45). Clinical neuropsychology. Amsterdam: Elsevier Science Publishers; 1985. p. 205–18.

Daniel BT. Transient global amnesia. Print version and ebook: Amazon; 2012.

Faust JS, Nemes A. Transient global amnesia: emergency department evaluation and management. Emerg Med Pract. 2016;18:1–20.

Forman WB. Transient global amnesia: a case report and literature review. Am J Hosp Palliat Care. 2012;29:563–5.

Griebe M, Bäzner H, Kablau M, Hennerici MG, Szabo K. Transient global amnesia in legal proceedings. Int J Legal Med. 2015;129:223–6.

Harrison M, Williams M. The diagnosis and management of transient global amnesia in the emergency department. Emerg Med J. 2007;24:444–5.

Hodges JR. Transient amnesia. Clinical and neuropsychological aspects. London: WB Saunders; 1991.

Hunter G. Transient global amnesia. Neurol Clin. 2011;29:1045-54.

Kirshner HS. Transient global amnesia: a brief review and update. Curr Neurol Neurosci Rep. 2011;11:578-82.

Klötzsch C. Transient global amnesia: diagnosis and differential diagnosis [in German]. Fortschr Neurol Psychiatr. 2009;77:669-77.

Kritchevsky M. Transient global amnesia. In: Squire LR, Butters N, editors. Neuropsychology of memory. 2nd ed. New York: Guilford Press; 1992. p. 147–55

Larner AJ. Neuropsychological neurology: the neurocognitive impairments of neurological disorders. Cambridge: Cambridge University Press; 2008a. p. 114.

Larner AJ. Transient acute neurologic sequelae of sexual activity: headache and amnesia. J Sex Med. 2008b;5:284–8.

Larner AJ. Neuropsychological neurology: the neurocognitive impairments of neurological disorders. 2nd ed. Cambridge: Cambridge University Press; 2013. p. 88.

Larner AJ. Dementia in clinical practice: a neurological perspective. Pragmatic studies in the cognitive function clinic. 2nd ed. London: Springer; 2014.

Larner AJ, Coles AJ, Scolding NJ, Barker RA. A-Z of neurological practice. A guide to clinical neurology. 2nd ed. London: Springer; 2011. p. 734–5.

Marazzi C, Scoditti U, Ticinesi A et al. Transient global amnesia. Acta Biomed. 2014;85:229-35.

Marin-Garcia E, Ruiz-Vargas JM. Transient global amnesia: a review. I. Clinical aspects [in Spanish]. Rev Neurol. 2008;46:53–60.

Markowitsch HJ, editor. Transient global amnesia and related disorders. Toronto: Hogrefe and Huber; 1990.

Owen D, Paranandi B, Sivakumar R, Seevaratnam M. Classical diseases revisited: transient global amnesia. Postgrad Med J. 2007;83:236-9.

Quinette P, Guillery-Girard B, Dayan J, de la Sayette V, Marquis S, Viader F, Desgranges B, Eustache F. What does transient global amnesia really mean? Review of the literature and thorough study of 142 cases. Brain 2006;129:1640-58.

Sander K, Sander D. New insights into transient global amnesia: recent imaging and clinical findings. Lancet Neurol. 2005;4:437-44.

Shekhar R. Transient global amnesia—a review. Int J Clin Pract. 2008;62:939-42.

Simos PG, Papanicolaou AC. Transient global amnesia. In: Papanicolaou AC. The amnesias: a clinical textbook of memory disorders. Oxford: Oxford University Press; 2006. p. 171-89.

Szabo K. Transient global amnesia. In: Szabo K, Hennerici MG, editors. The hippocampus in clinical neuroscience. Basel: Karger; 2014. p. 143–9.

Urban PP. Paroxysmal memory loss. In: Schmitz B, Tettenborn B, Schomer DL, editors. The paroxysmal disorders. Cambridge: Cambridge University Press; 2010. p. 158-63.

Veran O, Barre M, Casez O, Vercueil L. Idiopathic transient global amnesia [in French]. Psychol Neuropsychiatr Vieil. 2008;6:265-75.

Whitty CWM. Transient global amnesia. In: Whitty CWM, Zangwill OL, editors. Amnesia. Clinical, psychological and medicolegal aspects. 2nd ed. London: Butterworths; 1977. p. 93–103.

Wilkinson T, Derry C. Transient global amnesia. Pulse. 2014;25 November: http://www.pulsetoday.co.uk/confirmation?rtn=http://www.pulsetoday.co.uk/clinical/neurology-clinic-transient-global-amnesia/20008557.article.

Williamson J, Larner AJ. Transient global amnesia. Br J Hosp Med. 2015;76:C186-8.

Zeman AZ, Hodges JR. Transient global amnesia. Br J Hosp Med. 1997;58:257-60.

Preface to the Second Edition [2022]

This new edition encompasses 20 years of personal experience in seeing TGA patients, incorporates much new material on TGA published in the last 5 years, and also includes some old material previously missed or overlooked. Whilst reviews of TGA continue to appear [1, 2], the more significant development has been in the number of systematic reviews, meta-analyses, and studies using population-based datasets which have begun to emerge.

Whilst the arrangement of the chapters in this edition remains unchanged, those on investigation and epidemiology have both been split into two chapters to make them less unwieldy, the former because of the significant increase in the number of neuroimaging studies of TGA. As in the first edition, the purpose has not been to attempt to catalogue every single paper ever published on the subject but to elucidate key themes as currently understood.

The most significant change has been the attempt to develop more on the pathogenic mechanisms of TGA, beyond the traditional stroke/epilepsy/migraine concepts (Chap. 9). Admittedly this is more speculative than, although developed from, the evidence base described in the rest of the book, but the absence of any particular TGA hypothesis was an acknowledged lacuna in the first edition.

Liverpool, UK   A.J. Larner

References

1. Nehring SM, Spurling BC, Kumar A. Transient global amnesia. In: StatPearls [Internet]. Treasure Island, FL: StatPearls Publishing; 2021.
2. Spiegel DR, Smith J, Wade RR et al. Transient global amnesia: current perspectives. Neuropsychiatr Dis Treatment. 2017;13:2691–703.

Acknowledgements

As before, thanks are due to the many colleagues from whom I have learned much, both directly and indirectly about TGA, including Mark Doran, Rhys Davies (both in Liverpool), John Hodges, Adam Zeman, and Chris Butler.

My thanks are also due to Elizabeth Larner for producing many of the figures (2.1, 2.2, 9.1, 9.2, 9.3, and 9.5).

All errors or misconceptions which remain are entirely my own work.

AJ Larner MD PhD FRCP
Cognitive Function Clinic
Walton Centre for Neurology and Neurosurgery
Lower Lane
Fazakerley
Liverpool
L9 7LJ
United Kingdom
e-mail: andrew.larner2@nhs.net

Contents

Chapter 1
History of TGA

Abstract This chapter considers the history of TGA. This may be dated from the first use of the term "transient global amnesia" by Fisher and Adams in their publications of 1958 and 1964, but the characteristic clinical features had been described earlier than this under different appellations, in both the English ("episode of confusion with amnesia") and French ("les ictus amnésiques") literature. To date, the earliest probable case noted is that published by Benon in 1909. The reports retrospectively identified as suggestive of TGA had already described the associations with catheter angiography of the vertebral arteries and with migraine.

Keywords TGA · History

1.1 Beginnings: Fisher and Adams' First Accounts of TGA

The syndrome of transient global amnesia (TGA) was first described as such by the neurologists C. Miller Fisher (1913–2012) and Raymond D. Adams (1911–2008) in 1958 [1] and 1964 [2].

In an interview with Raymond Adams, his biographer Robert Laureno asked him whether he recalled any of his cases:

> RA: Our first case was the wife of the dean of a medical school, who brought her to me. They had been at their summer place. It was their practice to get up in the morning to go for a swim in the cold north shore water. She set the breakfast table. When they returned from the swim, she had no memory of having set the table or having gone for the swim. Her memory for the day before was virtually nil. He called me and brought her to the Massachusetts General Hospital that afternoon and by then she was completely recovered. She did not remember the episode or the events of the preceding hours. That was our first case, several years before our publication ([3], p.107).

In their first published report, of 1958, Fisher and Adams described 12 cases with a relatively uniform and stereotyped clinical picture consisting of a profound but transient amnesic syndrome which they believed had not previously been described in the medical literature and which they called "transient global amnesia" [1]. Only

© The Author(s), under exclusive license to Springer Nature
Switzerland AG 2022
A.J. Larner, *Transient Global Amnesia*,
https://doi.org/10.1007/978-3-030-98939-2_1

1

later did it become apparent that not all mnestic function is impaired in transient global amnesia (see Chap. 2 and Sect. 4.1.1) and hence that "global" may be a misnomer. At the time of this publication, the deeper fractionation of mnestic processes, much of it related to work on patient HM [4], had not yet impacted clinical practice.

Fisher and Adams' subsequent paper, published in 1964, was an altogether more substantial affair, indeed comprising an entire supplement of the journal *Acta Neurologica Scandinavica*. This was an amplification of the earlier paper, now presenting 17 extensive case descriptions as well as discussions of the possible aetiology of TGA, of which their favoured explanation, albeit tentative, was "a special type of focal cerebral seizure" [2]. Caplan's biography of Fisher adds no other details about these inaugural TGA papers [5].

TGA represents just one of Raymond Adams' many major contributions in neurology, as listed in Laureno's biography [3]. However, whether this could be labelled as an "original" contribution is moot. Although new neurological diseases do sometimes emerge, it would seem a priori that TGA was not a new condition when Fisher and Adams described it, contrary to their statement that it "appeared to represent a distinct clinical syndrome which heretofore had not been delineated in the literature" [2]. Indeed, prior reports documenting cases similar to, and almost certainly representing examples of, what Fisher and Adams called TGA (and of which they were apparently unaware) may also be found in the literature, accounts which might be figuratively termed the "prehistory" of TGA.

1.2   "Prehistory" of TGA

In 1956, Morris Bender described 12 patients who experienced an "isolated episode of confusion with amnesia", which was characterised by a "single brief period of defective memory and confusion with a complete retrograde amnesia". Repetition of the same questions by the patient was a frequent clinical observation. Attacks were reported to last for a few hours but did not recur. Bender found it difficult to classify these events, but favoured a "transient circulatory disturbance of the brain" [6]. A later paper by the same author detailed the clinical features in 26 patients and emphasised the absence of recurrence [7]. Jaffe and Bender subsequently reported on 51 patients, with particular reference to electroencephalographic (EEG) findings [8] (Sect. 4.2.1).

Contemporaneously with Bender's first (1956) account, though the authors were evidently unknown to one another, Guyotat and Courjon writing in the French literature described 16 patients with "l'ictus amnésique" [9], a syndrome of "transient loss of retrograde memory without diffuse loss of brain function" (translation of Pearce and Bogousslavasky; [10], p.189). In contrast to Bender's report, six of their sixteen patients had more than one episode. The possibility of recurrence of amnesic attacks was subsequently also mentioned by Fisher and Adams [2].

Prior to Guyotat and Courjon [9], the term "ictus amnésique" had been in use, apparently originating with Jean Alfred Fournier in 1879 who reported patients with amnesic spells in the context of tabes and general paresis ([10], p.188). The term was also subsequently used to describe other cases which appeared in the French literature which are likely to have been examples of TGA ([11], p.3).

In 1954, Hauge described three cases of acute and transient memory loss following catheter angiography of the vertebral arteries. Some patients had visual disturbances which resembled migraine following the injection of contrast media [12]. Retrospectively, it seems likely that these cases probably correspond with what Fisher and Adams called TGA. Other cases of TGA associated with angiographic procedures have subsequently been described (see Sect. 3.1.5 and Table 3.6).

When John Hodges published his influential monograph on TGA in 1991, it was thought that Hauge's account was probably the earliest description of TGA ([11], p.3). Hodges did note, however, that earlier cases of TGA might have been "immersed in the literature on psychogenic amnesia" ([11], p.4) and cited possible examples from the 1939 publication of Kanzer [13]. Hodges noted the concurrent decrease in reports of "hysterical amnesia" and increase in reports of TGA from the 1960s onwards. Gil et al. later challenged Hodges' contention, finding a "clear differentiation between hysterical amnesia and amnesia triggered by an emotional shock" in the 1900 textbook of Paul Sollier (1861–1933), a student of Charcot, dating from the late nineteenth century [14]. Gil et al. also state that Sollier's 1900 book portrayed "characteristic descriptions of transient global amnesia after a violent emotional shock" [14].

However, the earliest report which, at time of writing, seems to be acknowledged as likely to be a typical case of TGA, as noted by Berrios ([15], p.22), is that presented by R Benon in 1909, under the rubric of "ictus amnésique" [16]. Of the four patients reported, one ("*Observation II*") documented a 66-year-old woman who had an episode lasting 4–5 h characterised by an amnesic state with repetitive questioning, a retrograde amnesia of at least 30 years, but without other neurological signs (see the translation in Pearce and Bogousslavsky's paper [10] which commemorates the 100th anniversary of Benon's publication). There was no recurrence during a 3-year period of follow-up. Benon drew a distinction between these cases of "organic" amnesia and those which occurred in the context of general paresis (syphilis) on which he had published previously [17].

Daniel ([18], p.2) states that the French clinician Théodule-Armand Ribot (1839–1916) "described transient amnestic states suggestive of TGA" in his 1881 volume on *Disorders of Memory*. This claim for the priority of Ribot has also been made by other authors writing on TGA [19, 20], but likewise eschewing quotation or precise page citation from Ribot's book. Consulting the English translation of the book made by William Huntington Smith and published in New York in 1882 [21], Ribot certainly addresses the subject of temporary amnesia, as compared with periodic and progressive amnesia. The most suggestive account is simply a citation ([21], pp. 123–7) of a case previously presented in 1835 by "Kömpfen" [22] which followed a head injury, an exclusion criterion for TGA (see Sect. 2.2.2). Hence, I find no compelling account of TGA in Ribot [23], contrary to previous claims to that effect [18–20].

Berrios claims descriptions of transient global amnesia in the works of Jules Falret (1865) ([15], p.18) and Forbes Winslow (1861) ([15], p.16, 22). In the latter's *On obscure diseases of the brain and disorders of the mind*, in the chapter (XIV) devoted to "Acute disorders of the memory" [24], I find no account suggestive of TGA (Berrios [15], p.22, quotes from this chapter, but his page citation, p.372, is incorrect; the quote is from p.342). Trimble states that "In the nineteenth century … examples of what we now refer to as transient global amnesia were reported" but gives no references ([25], p.176–7).

This is not to say, of course, that TGA did not occur before the twentieth century: absence of evidence is not equivalent to evidence of absence. The ontological challenge to the persistence of disease over historical time, suggesting as it does in this situation that mechanisms of mnestic hippocampal function have changed, is simply not credible [23].

1.3   After Fisher and Adams

It is acknowledged that TGA achieved general recognition as a distinct neurological condition after the term was introduced by Fisher and Adams ([10], p. 188), but this recognition was not achieved immediately.

Poser and Ziegler in 1960 reported cases of temporary amnesia which they ascribed to "cerebrovascular insufficiency" [26]. Despite the brevity of their clinical descriptions, Hodges ([11], p. 3) was "almost certain" that these represented cases of TGA. Amongst these were patients with an existing diagnosis of migraine (see Sect. 3.4.1 and Sect. 7.9), probably the first report of the concurrence of these conditions. (Incidentally, Poser did later adopt the term "transient global amnesia", although the patient reported under this nomenclature had memory problems for several days [27]. Nevertheless, Caplan included this case in his 1985 literature review [28].) The possible link between TGA and migraine was later emphasised by Caplan et al. in 1981 [29].

Evans in 1966 reported three patients with transient loss of memory, of whom two had attacks suggestive of TGA in the context of a history of migraine. The third patient had a history of temporal lobe epilepsy and the reported attack lasted more than 48 hours so is unlikely to have been TGA [30]. Another early report was that of Bolwig, in 1968, who presented four cases and favoured "transient ischemia in the hippocampal region" as the aetiological explanation [31].

Recurrence of TGA attacks, although previously mentioned in the literature, for example, by Guyotat and Courjon [9] and by Fisher and Adams [2], was made explicit by Lou [32] (Sect. 6.2), although at least one patient in this series almost certainly had an ischaemic aetiology (see Sect. 3.1).

Just as early accounts of patients with what would now be called TGA may be found in the literature on psychogenic amnesia ([11], p.4), it is also possible that some cases labelled as having Korsakoff's syndrome might in fact be examples of TGA. From 1887 onwards, Sergei Korsakoff described cases of dense anterograde amnesia in alcoholic patients, although earlier accounts had appeared, for example, that of Robert Lawson in 1878 [33, 34]. Reports of "transient Korsakoff's syndrome" but with clinical details suggestive of TGA may be found in the literature, predating the widespread awareness of the TGA construct [35, 36].

An example of the increased recognition of the condition, and the ascendancy of Fisher and Adams' proposed TGA nomenclature, was provided by the consecutive editions of Whitty and Zangwill's textbook devoted to the subject of amnesia. In the first edition of 1966, Whitty and Lishman, in their chapter entitled "Amnesia in cerebral disease", mentioned only Fisher and Adams' original 1958 paper, under the subheading of "Transient vascular occlusions" ([37], p.51). However, by the time of the second edition of the book, published in 1977, a whole chapter was devoted exclusively to TGA, including a case personally observed by Whitty [38].

During this period, cases of TGA also began to be reported in languages other than English (e.g. [39–42]). Perhaps the first monograph on the subject was published by Gerhard Frank in 1981, reporting 27 personally observed cases [43].

An issue that emerged with these early reports, particularly noted in retrospect, related to exactly what qualified for inclusion as "TGA" as conceptualised by Fisher and Adams, and what did not, what was distinct and hence possibly a different disorder or disorders. In other words, the term "TGA" might have been applied somewhat loosely in these early accounts. By the time of Caplan's 1985 review [28], he was able to present data relating to 485 TGA patients reported in the literature and suggested some boundaries for inclusion and exclusion (see Sect. 2.2.1). This trend inevitably culminated in the formulation of diagnostic criteria for TGA, proposed by Hodges and Warlow in 1990 [44], based on their clinico-epidemiological study of TGA (Sect. 2.2.2). These proposals were somewhat more stringent than Caplan's proposed inclusion/exclusion boundaries.

These developments coincided with the advent of the widespread availability of neuroimaging techniques, initially computed tomography (CT), in neurological practice. Although CT contributed rather little to the understanding of TGA (Sect. 5.1.1), it was the harbinger of the rapid development in neuroimaging techniques, particularly magnetic resonance imaging, which has contributed to understanding of the condition and which will be discussed later in greater detail (Sect. 5.1.2).

The volume devoted largely to TGA which was edited by Markowitsch in 1990 [45] and the monograph by Hodges published in 1991 [11], the latter based on the seminal publications of the Oxford TGA study (e.g. [44, 46–48]), indicated that TGA had become a widely recognised condition and a legitimate subject for ongoing investigations. Since then, Hodges and Warlow's diagnostic criteria [44] have been increasingly applied to TGA case definition. Retrospectively, there may be caveats regarding cases labelled as "TGA" which were described prior to the adoption of these criteria (e.g. see specific cases in the series reported by Evans [30] and Lou [32], as mentioned above).

Notable contributions in more recent years have been the extensive review by Quinette et al. in 2006 of 142 personally observed cases and 1353 cases found in the literature [49]. Daniel (2012) reviewed several hundred publications related to TGA in his book [18], to my knowledge the most recent book length publication devoted exclusively to TGA prior to the first edition of this book published in 2017. Recourse to a PubMed search using the title words "transient global amnesia" returned 668 hits to the end of 2016 (accessed 02/01/2017) and 830 hits to the end of 2021 (accessed 31/12/21). This is certainly an underestimate of all publications related to TGA, since papers describing cases do not necessarily have this term in the title (Sect. 1.4). Of these articles, major series and systematic studies have until recent times been relatively few (e.g. [50, 51], most publications reporting only single or a few cases.

1.4   A Note on Nomenclature

As well as "ictus amnésiques" [9], a number of other terms have been used on occasion to describe what appear to be typical TGA episodes. These include:

- episodic global amnesia (by Adams, cited in Laureno [3], p.145). This may owe something to the terminology of "episode(s) of confusion with amnesia" used by Bender [6, 7] and Jaffe and Bender [8].
- amnestic episodes (e.g. [39, 52], perhaps related to the appellation in German ("Amnestische Episoden", e.g. [43]).
- transitory global amnesia (e.g. [39, 53–55], perhaps related to the appellations in French ("amnesia global transitoire", e.g. [56]) and Spanish ("amnesia global transitoria" or AGT, e.g. [57]).
- paroxysmal memory loss [58].

In this text, the familiar "transient global amnesia" terminology coined by Fisher and Adams [1, 2] will be used throughout.

1.5   A Note on Methodology

Because TGA is a relatively rare condition, the majority of publications have been single case reports or small case series. This anecdotal, opportunistic and unsystematic literature constitutes the lowest rung on the ladder of clinical evidence (e.g. [59, 60]) and has been previously criticised [48]. Although this evidence is not ignored here, the findings may be less robust than those emerging from case–control studies, population cohort studies (e.g. [50, 51]), systematic reviews (e.g. [61]) and meta-analyses (e.g. [62, 63]). These studies are far less common, but will be emphasised in this text.

1.6 Summary and Recommendations

Although first described as such in the late 1950s and early 1960s, the syndrome of transient global amnesia has probably been reported in the medical literature under other nomenclature since the beginning of the twentieth century. It would seem likely that the human brain has always been vulnerable to this syndrome.

References

1. Fisher CM, Adams RD. Transient global amnesia. Trans Am Neurol Assoc. 1958;83:143–6.
2. Fisher CM, Adams RD. Transient global amnesia. Acta Neurol Scand. 1964;40(Suppl9):1–81.
3. Raymond Adams LR. A life of mind and muscle. Oxford: Oxford University Press, 2009. p. 106–7. 145,187,191
4. Scoville WB, Milner B. Loss of recent memory after bilateral hippocampal lesions. J Neurol Neurosurg Psychiatry. 1957;30:11–21.
5. Caplan LR, Miller Fisher C. Stroke in the 20th century. New York: Oxford University Press; 2020.
6. Bender MB. Syndrome of isolated episode of confusion with amnesia. J Hillside Hosp. 1956;5:212–5.
7. Bender MB. Single episode of confusion with amnesia. Bull NY Acad Med. 1960;36:197–207.
8. Jaffe R, Bender MB. E.E.G. studies in the syndrome of isolated episodes of confusion with amnesia "transient global amnesia". J Neurol Neurosurg Psychiatry. 1966;29:472–4.
9. Guyotat MM, Courjon J. Les ictus amnésiques. J Med Lyon. 1956;37:697–701.
10. Pearce JMS, Bogousslavsky J. "Les ictus amnésiques" and transient global amnesia. Eur Neurol. 2009;62:188–92.
11. Hodges JR. Transient amnesia. Clinical and neuropsychological aspects. London: WB Saunders; 1991.
12. Hauge T. Catheter vertebral angiography. Acta Radiol Suppl. 1954;109:1–219.
13. Kanzer M. Amnesia. A statistical study. Am J Psychiatry. 1939;96:711–6.
14. Gil R, Abdul-Samad F, Mathis S, Neau JP. Was there a confusion before 1950 between global transient global [sic] amnesia and psychogenic amnesia? [in French]. Rev Neurol (Paris). 2010;166:699–703.
15. Berrios GE. Historical aspects of memory and its disorders. In: Berrios GE, Hodges JR, editors. Memory disorders in psychiatric practice. Cambridge: Cambridge University Press; 2000. p. 3–33.
16. Benon R. Les ictus amnésiques dans les démences "organiques". Ann Méd Psychol. 1909;67:207–19.
17. Benon R. Les ictus amnésiques dans la paralysie générale. Gaz Hôp (Paris). 1908;1335
18. Daniel BT. Transient global amnesia. Print version and ebook: Amazon; 2012.
19. Foss-Skiftesvik J, Snoer AH, Wagner A, Hauerberg J. Transient global amnesia after cerebral angiography still occurs: case report and literature review. Radiol Case Rep. 2015;9:988.
20. Hunter G. Transient global amnesia. Neurol Clin. 2011;29:1045–54.
21. Ribot T. Diseases of memory: an essay in the positive psychology. New York: D Appleton and Company; 1882. https://archive.org/stream/cu31924031165719?ref=ol#page/n39/mode/2up
22. Koempfen M. Observation sur un cas de perte de mémoire. Mémoires de l'Academie Nationale de Médecine. 1835;4:489–94. https://gallica.bnf.fr/ark:/12148/bpt6k6361350t/f507.item
23. Larner AJ. Did Ribot describe transient global amnesia in the nineteenth century? Cortex. 2021;138:38–9.

24. Winslow F. On obscure diseases of the brain and disorders of the mind. London: John W Davies; 1861. https://www.google.co.uk/books/edition/On_obscure_diseases_of_the_Brain_and_dis/X3taAAAAcAAJ?hl=en&gbpv=1&printsec=frontcover
25. Trimble MR. The intentional brain. Motion, emotion, and the development of modern neuropsychiatry. Baltimore: Johns Hopkins University Press; 2016.
26. Poser CM, Ziegler DK. Temporary amnesia as a manifestation of cerebrovascular insufficiency. Trans Am Neurol Assoc. 1960;85:221–3.
27. Roman-Campos G, Poser CM, Wood FB. Persistent retrograde memory deficit after transient global amnesia. Cortex. 1980;16:509–18.
28. Caplan LB. [sic]. Transient global amnesia. In: Frederiks JAM, editor. Handbook of clinical neurology. Volume 1 (45). Clinical neuropsychology. Amsterdam: Elsevier Science Publishers; 1985. p. 205–18.
29. Caplan L, Chedru F, Lhermitte F, Mayman C. Transient global amnesia and migraine. Neurology. 1981;31:1167–70.
30. Evans JH. Transient loss of memory, an organic mental syndrome. Brain. 1966;89:539–48.
31. Bolwig TG. Transient global amnesia. Acta Neurol Scand. 1968;44:101–6.
32. Lou H. Repeated episodes of transient global amnesia. Acta Neurol Scand. 1968;44:612–8.
33. Larner AJ, Gardner-Thorpe C. Robert Lawson (?1846-1896). J Neurol. 2012;259:792–3.
34. Lawson R. On the symptomatology of alcoholic brain disorders. Brain. 1878;1:182–94.
35. Deak G, Toth S. Vertebral angiography followed by transient Korsakoff's syndrome [in Hungarian]. Ideggyogy Sz. 1964;17:119–25.
36. de Tribolet N, Assal G, Oberson R. Korsakoff's syndrome and transitory cortical blindness following vertebral angiography [in German]. Schweiz Med Wochenschr. 1975;105:1506–9.
37. Whitty CWM, Lishman WA. Amnesia in cerebral disease. In: Whitty CWM, Zangwill OL, editors. Amnesia. London: Butterworths; 1966. p. 36–76.
38. Whitty CWM. Transient global amnesia. In: Whitty CWM, Zangwill OL, editors. Amnesia. Clinical, psychological and medicolegal aspects. 2nd ed. London: Butterworths; 1977. p. 93–103.
39. Flügel KA. Syndrome of transitory global amnesia (amnestic episodes) [in German]. Fortschr Med. 1974;92:1067–71.
40. Frank G. Clinical observations on the psychopathology of amnesic episodes (transient global amnesia) (author's transl.) [in German]. Arch Psychiatr Nervenkr (1970). 1976;223:89–98.
41. Godlewski S. Amnesic episodes (transient global amnesia). (Clinical study based on 33 unpublished cases) [in French]. Sem Hop. 1968;44:553–77.
42. Müller D. Amnestic episodes. (Isolated episodes of confusion with amnesia, amnesic ictus, transient global amnesia) [in Greek, Modern]. Psychiatr Neurol Med Psychol (Leipz). 1975;27:463–9.
43. Frank G. Amnestische Episoden. Berlin: Springer-Verlag; 1981.
44. Hodges JR, Warlow CP. Syndromes of transient amnesia: towards a classification. A study of 153 cases. J Neurol Neurosurg Psychiatry. 1990;53:834–43.
45. Markowitsch HJ, editor. Transient global amnesia and related disorders. Toronto: Hogrefe and Huber; 1990.
46. Hodges JR, Oxbury SM. Persistent memory impairment following transient global amnesia. J Clin Exp Neuropsychol. 1990;12:904–20.
47. Hodges JR, Ward CD. Observations during transient global amnesia. A behavioural and neuropsychological study of five cases. Brain. 1989;112:595–620.
48. Hodges JR, Warlow CP. The aetiology of transient global amnesia. A case-control study of 114 cases with prospective follow-up. Brain. 1990;113:639–57.
49. Quinette P, Guillery-Girard B, Dayan J, de la Sayette V, Marquis S, Viader F, Desgranges B, Eustache F. What does transient global amnesia really mean? Review of the literature and thorough study of 142 cases. Brain. 2006;129:1640–58.
50. Lin KH, Chen YT, Fuh JL, et al. Migraine is associated with a higher risk of transient global amnesia: a nationwide cohort study. Eur J Neurol. 2014;21:718–24.

51. Yi M, Sherzai AZ, Ani C, Shavlik D, Ghamsary M, Lazar E, Sherzai D. Strong association between migraine and transient global amnesia: a national inpatient sample analysis. J Neuropsychiatry Clin Neurosci. 2019;31:43–8.
52. Mumenthaler M, Treig T. Amnestic episodes. Analysis of 111 personal cases. [in German]. Schweiz Med Wochenschr. 1984;114:1163–70.
53. Maggioni F, Mainardi F, Bellamio M, Zanchin G. Transient global amnesia triggered by migraine in monozygotic twins. Headache. 2011;51:1305–8.
54. Pillmann F, Broich K. Transitory global amnesia—psychogenic origin of organic disease? Psychopathologic basis and pathogenetic considerations [in German]. Fortschr Neurol Psychiatr. 1998;66:160–3.
55. Toledo M, Pujadas F, Purroy F, Alvarez-Sabin J. Polycythaemia as a ready factor of transitory global amnesia [in Spanish]. Neurologia. 2005;20:317–20.
56. Boudin G, Pépin B, Mikol J, Haguenau M, Vernant JC. Gliome du systeme limbique posterieur, revele par une amnesia globale transitoire. Observation anatomo-clinique d'un cas. Rev Neurol. 1975;131:157–63.
57. Riva C, Leiva C, Gobernado JM, Gimeno A. Amnesia global transitoria asociada a un meningioma del lobulo frontal. Med Clin (Barc). 1985;84:81.
58. Urban PP. Paroxysmal memory loss. In: Schmitz B, Tettenborn B, Schomer DL, editors. The paroxysmal disorders. Cambridge: Cambridge University Press; 2010. p. 158–63.
59. Brainin M, Barnes M, Baron JC, et al. Guidance for the preparation of neurological management guidelines by EFNS scientific task forces – revised recommendations 2004. Eur J Neurol. 2004;11:577–81.
60. Leone MA, Brainin M, Boon P, et al. Guidance for the preparation of neurological management guidelines by EFNS scientific task forces—revised recommendations 2012. Eur J Neurol. 2013;20:410–9.
61. Milburn-McNulty P, Larner AJ. Transient global amnesia and brain tumour: chance concurrence or aetiological association? Case report and systematic literature review. Case Rep Neurol. 2015;7:18–25.
62. Jäger T, Bazner H, Kliegel M, Szabo K, Hennerici MG. The transience and nature of cognitive impairments in transient global amnesia: a meta-analysis. J Clin Exp Neuropsychol. 2009;31:8–19.
63. Modabbernia A, Taslimi S, Ashrafi M, Modabbernia MJ, Hu HH. Internal jugular vein reflux in patients with transient global amnesia: a meta-analysis of case-control studies. Acta Neurol Belg. 2012;112:237–44.

Chapter 2
Clinical Features, Diagnostic Criteria and Possible Variants of TGA

Abstract This chapter begins with a consideration of the typical clinical features of an attack of TGA. Although relatively stereotyped, nevertheless different authors have used the "TGA" terminology to describe different events characterised by transient amnesia. Following the description of possible boundaries for what might be included or excluded from the TGA label, diagnostic criteria were developed by Hodges and Warlow in 1990 for definite or pure TGA. Whether variants of TGA exist is still uncertain; if so, they are much rarer, gauged by the frequency of published reports.

Keywords TGA · Clinical features · Diagnostic criteria · Variants

2.1 Clinical Features of TGA

2.1.1 TGA Archetype

The clinical features of transient global amnesia (TGA) are best illustrated by citing a typical case history, and it is generally acknowledged that in this regard the descriptions by Fisher and Adams [1, 2] are archetypal:

Case 1. Man, aged 67

The patient, a brilliant professional man, suffered his attack immediately after he had spent about one and a half hours being interviewed by two journalists at his home. The subject of the discussion was the history of an organization some 33 years ago and the details provided proved accurate and during the interview the journalists noted no abnormality in the patient whatsoever. As the visitors left, the patient bade them goodby [sic] and added a few appropriately humorous words. The members of his family were standing in the hallway 15 to 20 feet away and the patient was in full view and earshot while the visitors were leaving. The patient turned and walked towards his family, not saying anything but looking puzzled. He then asked, "Who are they?" (the visitors), "What are they doing here?" [.] Then he asked how it happened that certain members of his family were present (they had come for a visit the previous day). Then he asked if the family noticed anything wrong with him. The patient was quite worried and clearly appreciated that he could not

A.J. Larner, *Transient Global Amnesia*, https://doi.org/10.1007/978-3-030-98939-2_2

11

remember and could not collect his thoughts (one of the family members present was a physician and provided most of the details of the events). For the next hour or hour and a half the patient repeatedly asked somewhat similar questions: "Who was that? What were they doing here? What are you doing here? Do you see anything wrong with me?"[.] As each question was answered he would go on to another, so that the repetition was not wholly automatic. But if he remained quiet for a minute or so he would again begin a repetition of the same questions. There was no dysarthria or dysphasia ([2], p.9).

The typical features of TGA, made evident not only by the accounts of Fisher and Adams by also by earlier authors [3, 4], consist of an abrupt attack of impaired antcrograde memory, affecting both verbal and non-verbal components, often manifest as repeated, iterative, circular, questioning, but without clouding of consciousness or focal neurological signs. The questions are usually of a self-orienting nature (e.g. Where am I? What is happening?). Also evident from clinical observation is concurrent retrograde amnesia of variable duration, whereas personal identification and other aspects of memory (working memory, semantic memory, implicit memory) appear to be intact (see Sect. 4.1 for more detailed discussion of the neuropsychological features of TGA).

Patient behaviour during an attack is also characteristic. The insight that something is wrong is not uncommon [5], with the patient manifesting a sense of bewilderment or perplexity to onlookers, sometimes amounting to agitation or distress, although sometimes the affect is rather flattened.

2.1.2   Accompanying Neurological and Psychological Symptoms

Neurological symptoms during an attack may include a complaint of headache (sometimes consistent with migraine), nausea and vomiting, and sometimes dizziness and sleepiness. For example, in a series of 203 episodes of TGA reported by Ahn et al. [6], the most common associated symptoms were headache (14.8%), dizziness (6.4%) and nausea/vomiting (5.4%). A wide variety of other symptoms has also been described on occasion, including chills/flushes, fear of dying (angor animi), paraesthesia, cold extremities, trembling, sweating, winding, and palpitations [7], suggestive of activation of the autonomic nervous system.

Focal neurological signs described in some of the early reports of "TGA" (e.g. dysarthria, dysphasia, visual field defects, hemiparesis) would now be considered to exclude the diagnosis of TGA (see Sect. 2.2). Subtle impairments of smooth pursuit eye movements have been documented using oculographic techniques within a median of 1 day of TGA episodes [8], but whether these are evident to unaided clinical neurological examination during attacks remains to be studied.

Acute changes in mood and anxiety levels have also been documented during TGA, the most common emotional symptoms being anxiety and depression. Inzitari et al. [9] noted symptoms during TGA were similar to those exhibited during a panic attack. A number of studies have subsequently documented symptoms of anxiety and depression during attacks by administering brief rating scales (respectively, the first part of the State-Trait Anxiety Inventory, and the Adjective Mood Scale or Befindlichkeits-Skala) [5, 10, 11]. Psychological factors may also be predisposing factors for TGA (Sect. 7.10).

2.1.3   Chronobiology: Diurnal Time of Onset

TGA attacks may occur at any time of the day. Diurnal variation in the time of onset, with attack onset most often in the morning or at midday, was reported in both a literature review ($n = 17$) and in a prospective patient cohort reported by Quinette et al. [7]. Attacks apparent on waking from sleep were not found, and indeed this may be an important differential diagnostic point, raising the possibility of an epileptic disorder (see Sect. 3.2 and Sect. 7.12). In the series of Ahn et al. [6], TGA episodes ($n = 203$) usually occurred in the morning (0600–1200 h: 36.5%) or in the afternoon (1200–1800 h: 38.9%). Oehler et al. reported one case "occurring exceptionally while sleeping" [12]. Hoyer et al., analysing data from two large TGA cohorts ($n = 404$ and 261, respectively), reported bimodal peaks of TGA occurrence at mid-morning and late afternoon in both cohorts, suggesting a robust circadian rhythm in TGA occurrence independent of patient gender and age [13].

Time of TGA onset by day of the week, month or season of the year is considered amongst predisposing factors of TGA (Sect. 7.2).

2.1.4   Attack Duration

Episodes of TGA are of brief duration, usually lasting between 1 and 10 h. The mean duration in two large series was 4.2 h [14] and 5.6 h [7]. In more recent series, Agosti et al. [15] reported the duration to be 4.3 ± 3.0 h, and Ahn et al. [6] reported a median duration of 5 h. Episodes lasting less than 1 h were previously considered rare (for example, Quinette et al. recorded only 3 such cases in 142 observed patients [7]) and potentially more suggestive of transient epileptic amnesia (Sect. 3.2). However, "short-duration TGA" (i.e. lasting <1 h) was noted to be quite common (8.8–32.0%) in three large independent cohort studies, with clinical features and long-term prognosis no different from longer episodes of TGA [16].

Because of the brevity of TGA, it is possible that many, if not most, attacks are not brought to medical attention. This has implications for attempts to quantitate disease incidence (Sect. 7.1). Extensive investigation post-event contributes relatively little information, but studies of neuropsychology, neurophysiology and neuroimaging during an attack have contributed to the understanding of TGA (see Chaps. 4 and 5).

2.1.5 Prognosis, Recurrence

The prognosis of TGA is generally excellent (see Chap. 6). There is usually an apparently complete recovery after the acute attack, aside from the absence of recollection for the amnesic period.

TGA attacks are usually solitary, but some patients experience recurrence (Sect. 6.2). Quoted recurrence rates may depend, of course, on the extent and completeness of patient follow-up, but the figure is probably around 5% [7]. A history of recurrent events may broaden the differential diagnosis (see Chap. 3), particularly the consideration of transient epileptic amnesia (Sect. 3.2; Case Study 2.1).

> **Case Study 2.1: Recurrent Attacks, Was it TGA?**
> A 60-year-old woman had experienced four episodes of transient amnesia over a 4-year period, all similar in form and all witnessed by her husband. All were associated with exercise (canoeing, cycling twice and swimming in cold water) and were characterised by repetitive questioning lasting between about 2 and 7 h with apparent complete recovery. Because of their recurrent nature, a provisional diagnosis of transient epileptic amnesia (TEA) had been made (MR brain imaging and EEG were both normal) and she was advised to stop driving and start taking an antiepileptic medication. She was not willing to contemplate medication so a second opinion was sought. On the basis of the witness account, the episodes were thought to be more typical of TGA than TEA, despite their recurrence. There were no episodes of amnesia on waking from sleep. On the Mini-Mental State Examination, she scored 30/30 and on the Montreal Cognitive Assessment 29/30. Over a 6-year period of follow-up, no further amnesic events occurred without antiepileptic drug treatment.

2.2   Diagnostic Criteria of TGA

2.2.1 Essential Features and Inclusion/Exclusion Boundaries

Although the clinical features of TGA are relatively stereotyped (Sect. 2.1), nevertheless episodes of transient amnesia may sometimes present diagnostic difficulties (see Chap. 3 for a consideration of the differential diagnosis). It should be remembered that not every paper purporting to describe TGA is necessarily describing TGA! To investigate a specific condition or disorder, in order to try to understand factors such as its epidemiology (see Chaps. 7 and 8) and pathogenesis (Chap. 9), it is obviously important that only examples of that disorder are examined and no other disorders which might seem clinically similar but which may have different causes. Hence the drive to codify clinical diagnosis by means of developing consensus diagnostic criteria, a project which has encompassed many neurological disorders (e.g. [17]). A similar rationale has been applied in TGA. As will be shown (see Chap. 3),

TGA has a potentially broad differential diagnosis, with a number of possible mimics or phenocopies.

Kane [18] recognised the need for diagnostic precision for TGA and listed ten "essential features" based on an experience of six patients followed up for 2.5 years, specifically:

- no premonitory transient ischaemic attack (TIA);
- risk factors for stroke often absent;
- isolated severe loss of recent memory (<24 h);
- complete clearing once episode is passed;
- patient aware/anxious about deficit;
- sparing of motor, visual and speech systems;
- no change in personality;
- persistence of unimpaired technical skills;
- rarely evolves to more characteristic stroke;
- rarely recurs ([18], p.726).

Perhaps implicit in these features was Kane's assumption that the pathology of TGA was vascular. Whilst these "essential features" have face validity, the definition of diagnostic criteria generally requires a more precise methodology and the examination of many more cases.

Caplan ([19], p.206–7) proposed "boundaries ... of what can be included within the diagnostic category of transient global amnesia, and what should properly be excluded", noting that hitherto such boundaries had been "fuzzy". The strict categorical definition of TGA which emerged was based on a large personal case series and literature review, with four points emerging as central to diagnosis, viz.:

1. "Information about the beginning of the attack should be available from a capable observer who witnessed the onset".

    This stipulation sought to exclude amnesic episodes secondary to trauma or epileptic seizure since these aetiologies could not be easily excluded if the onset of the event was unwitnessed.
2. "The patient should have been examined during the attack to be certain that other neurological symptoms and signs did not accompany the amnesia".

    The ideal of neurologist as examiner was noted to be impractical, since relatively few patients reach medical facilities within the time frame of an attack, and even if they do come to medical attention, clinicians with the skills and knowledge to undertake appropriate examination may not be immediately available. Caplan accepted that information from a "careful, concerned witness" who interacted with the patient would be acceptable, but patient self-report or information from casual companions would not.
3. "There should be no important accompanying neurological signs".
4. "The memory loss should be transient".

The extent of transience was not defined, and in his review, Caplan accepted cases of amnesia ranging in reported duration from 15 min to 7 days (cf. Sect. 2.1.4).

These "boundaries" defined by Caplan are still cited as "Diagnostic criteria for Transient Global Amnesia" in a textbook devoted to diagnostic criteria in neurology published in 2006 ([17], p.52–3) and certainly influenced subsequent thinking on the nature of TGA.

Of note, neither Kane nor Caplan appears to have been explicit about the exclusion of clouding or loss of consciousness in TGA, although this might be implicit in the formulation of "patient aware" [18] and "no … accompanying neurological signs" [19].

2.2.2   Hodges and Warlow's 1990 Diagnostic Criteria

Based upon their extensive clinical experience of TGA cases and a review of the literature, Hodges and Warlow [14] and Hodges ([20], p.6–12) developed seven diagnostic criteria for definite or pure TGA (see Table 2.1). These are explicit, inter alia, about level of consciousness and absence of aphasia.

(An eighth criterion was added by Nishiyama et al. [21], specifically for the diagnosis of transient partial verbal amnesia; see Sect. 2.3.2.)

The Hodges and Warlow 1990 criteria have become widely accepted and used (although, to my knowledge, have never been independently verified), indeed are now sometimes referred to as the "classical criteria" ([22], p.2270). Although the pre-1990 literature on TGA, predating the Hodges and Warlow criteria, will not be ignored in this book, post-1990 published material in which these diagnostic criteria have been applied will generally be given greater weight, as excluding other disorders which enter the differential diagnosis of TGA (see Chap. 3). Retrospectively, there may be caveats about some cases reported as "TGA" prior to the adoption of these criteria; re-analysis of the described clinical features may put some reports out with these diagnostic criteria. The "pure TGA" terminology had been used before

Table 2.1 Diagnostic criteria for definite TGA based on Hodges and Warlow 1990 [14] and Hodges 1991 ([20], p.12)

(a) Attacks must be witnessed and information available from a capable observer who was present for most of the attack.
(b) There must be clear-cut anterograde amnesia during the attack.
(c) Clouding of consciousness and loss of personal identity must be absent, and the cognitive impairment limited to amnesia (i.e. no aphasia, apraxia).
(d) There should be no accompanying focal neurological symptoms during the attack and no significant neurological signs afterwards.
(e) Epileptic features must be absent.
(f) Attacks must resolve within 24 h.
(g) Patients with recent head injury or active epilepsy (that is, remaining on medication or one seizure in the past two years) are excluded.

this landmark paper (e.g. [23, 24]) and has also been used on occasion since, specifically with respect to what might be termed "symptomatic" cases (e.g. [25–27]).

A reliable witness account of the attack is the first criterion; hence unwitnessed amnesic attacks cannot be diagnosed as TGA (e.g. Case Study 2.2). In their study of 153 cases of acute amnesia, Hodges and Warlow [14] excluded 39 cases (25%), the principal reason being unwitnessed attack ($n = 14$), followed by very limited details (8). In the author's personal series of acute amnesic patients seen over the period 2002–2021, 23 of 73 cases (31.5%) were excluded as not conforming to the Hodges and Warlow criteria (see also Fig. 7.3; note that these figures do not include cases confidently diagnosed as transient epileptic amnesia; Sect. 3.2).

> **Case Study 2.2: Unwitnessed Attack, Was it TGA?**
> A 79-year-old man was on a long walking expedition when he had an episode of impaired memory. No direct witness account was available, but apparently he had wanted to stop, had sat down and was asking repetitive questions for about half an hour. His wife attended the clinic with him but had not been with her husband on the walk, and by the time she had seen him several hours after the incident, he was apparently back to normal. A provisional diagnosis of TGA was made. (see Case Study 7.2 for further details.)

One implication emerging from the application of the Hodges and Warlow criteria is that diagnostic labels such as "TGA-like" syndrome (e.g. [28–33]) or "TGA-plus" syndrome (e.g. [34]) are misnomers. By applying the criteria, episodes are defined as "definite or pure TGA" or as "not TGA". To avoid potential confusion, a terminology that avoided the "TGA" label might be desirable to describe events not fulfilling TGA criteria: perhaps "transient amnesia of uncertain origin" or "transient amnesia not fulfilling criteria for TGA" would be preferable to "TGA-like" or "TGA-plus" syndromes.

The Hodges and Warlow criteria are entirely based on clinical history and examination findings, without recourse to any findings from investigations (see Chaps. 4 and 5). A corollary is that if the diagnosis of TGA is based on the use of these criteria then TGA remains a clinical diagnosis, with no current supplementary biomarkers (e.g. to help distinguish TGA from TEA). Whether the Hodges and Warlow criteria should be expanded in the light of more recent findings remains to be decided. For example, the possibility of modifying the criteria in the light of the neuroimaging changes observed in TGA, particularly diffusion-weighted magnetic resonance imaging sequences (Sect. 5.1.2), has been suggested (e.g. [35], p.109; [36]). The acute psychological changes (Sect. 2.1.2) are also overlooked by the Hodges and Warlow criteria, although "patient aware/anxious about deficit" was included amongst the ten "essential features" listed by Kane [18].

2.2.3 TGA Subtypes?

A question remaining unanswered by the Hodges and Warlow criteria is whether there might be subtypes of TGA, related to factors such as whether cases are idiopathic or symptomatic and whether episodes are single or recurrent.

A distinction may be drawn between a primary or idiopathic form of TGA and a secondary or symptomatic form of TGA, for example, TGA occurring secondary to a clear precipitating event, such as cerebral angiography (Sect. 3.1.6) or exposure to cold water (Sect. 1.1 and Sect. 8.3), or associated with a cerebral lesion such as an ischaemic stroke (Sect. 3.1.2) or tumour (Sect. 7.12). There is no evidence to suggest that these are different clinico-pathological entities, although whether the secondary or symptomatic forms shed any light on the pathogenesis of the primary or idiopathic form(s) remains to be established. The label of "spontaneous TGA" or "spontaneously occurring TGA" for those episodes occurring without an obvious precipitating factor is also questionable, as such factors may be identified with deeper analysis (Chap. 8).

At the time of Hodges and Warlow's studies, the only readily available neurological investigations included cerebrospinal fluid analysis, electroencephalography and brain imaging with computed tomography (CT) or single-photon emission computed tomography (SPECT). The greater spatial resolution of magnetic resonance (MR) brain imaging was not then easily accessed, let alone functional MR studies.

Agosti et al. [37] considered the validity of the Hodges and Warlow criteria in the light of a study of 130 consecutive patients with a first episode of TGA who underwent MR brain imaging, of whom 13 (10%) were found to have a structural brain lesion (leptomeningeal cysts 9; falx meningioma 2; cerebellar haemangioma 1; white matter hyperintensities in parieto-temporal region 1). In the light of these neuroradiological findings, they proposed that patients be classified into two subgroups, defined as primary TGA (classical attacks with normal neuroimaging: = TGA-p) and TGA patients with brain lesions (= TGA-b). No clinical or demographic differences were found between the two groups. This was perhaps not a surprising finding, since the brain lesions discovered on imaging were unlikely to be contributors to pathogenesis.

In a subsequent study, Agosti et al. [15] divided TGA patients (n = 243) according to whether or not they had evidence for internal jugular vein valve incompetence (IJVVI), a factor that was considered possibly relevant to TGA pathogenesis (Sect. 4.3.3.2 and Sect. 9.2.2). TGA patients with IJVVI showed a higher frequency of precipitating factors (Chap. 8) but had fewer vascular comorbidities (Sect. 7.11) than TGA patients without IJVVI, suggesting to these authors that there may be different mechanisms underpinning episodes of TGA.

Hence, it currently remains uncertain whether there is any merit in distinguishing TGA as either primary or secondary for the understanding of disease aetiology, although patient management in the latter category might be different. Investigations may disclose a symptomatic cause (e.g. the very rare instances of underlying

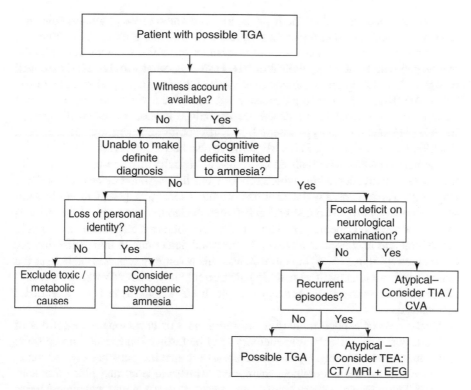

Fig. 2.1 Flow chart illustrating the possible decision-making process in the management of sus-pected TGA (adapted from [40])

multiple sclerosis [38, 39]) which may have distinct implications for patient treat-ment and management.

Another issue concerning TGA classification relates to recurrence. Although the annual recurrence rate is low (Sect. 6.2.1), some individuals do suffer recurrent TGA (e.g. Case Study 2.1), and there is some tentative evidence to suggest that these patients may differ in some respects from those with single episodes (Sect. 6.2.2), which might potentially impact on prognosis.

A flow chart illustrating the possible decision-making process in the manage-ment of suspected TGA is shown in Fig. 2.1.

2.3 Possible Variant Forms of TGA

TGA subgroups have been suggested on the basis of different precipitating events (see Chap. 8), namely physical exertion in men and emotional upset in women [7]. However, the possibility of distinct TGA phenotypic variants within the broad con-ceptualisation of TGA as an acute amnesic syndrome is considered here.

Alzheimer's disease (AD), perhaps the most common cause of amnesia encountered in clinical practice, typically presents as a syndrome of episodic amnesia, reflecting neuronal disconnection of hippocampal structures from the cortex by the plaque and tangle pathology typical of AD. However, other variants of AD are well recognised, resulting from pathological change predominating elsewhere in the brain [41]. Hence, logopenic progressive aphasia, visual variant/posterior cortical atrophy and even frontal variants are acknowledged in modern diagnostic criteria for AD [42], and a phenotype resembling corticobasal degeneration has also been described on occasion (e.g. [43]). Might there also be variant forms of TGA?

Memory may be conceptualised neuropsychologically as a non-uniform, distributed cognitive function within which subdivisions in function may be differentiated (Fig. 2.2), which involve various neuroanatomical substrates [44]. Current taxonomies of memory propose a distinction between declarative memory, also known as explicit or conscious memory, and non-declarative memory, also known as implicit, procedural and unconscious memory. Conceptual objections to this distinction are to be noted ([45], p.155–8), but nevertheless this taxonomy is presented here as the one most, if not all, cognitive neurologists current work with. "Working memory" or immediate memory is better conceptualised as an aspect of attentional mechanisms.

Declarative or explicit memories are intentional or conscious recollections of previous experience. Declarative memory may be further subdivided into episodic and semantic components. Episodic memories are specific personal events, sometimes known as autobiographical memories, which are time and place (context) specific. These may be either verbal or non-verbal (visual), with localising value to dominant and non-dominant hemispheres, respectively. Semantic memories, in contrast, are facts, a database of culturally-approved knowledge independent of any specific context. A distinction may also be drawn between anterograde memory, the laying down of new memories, and retrograde memory, the store of previously encoded material. Could any of these memory subsystems or subassemblies, whose anatomical substrates are thought to lie within the circuit of limbic structures proposed by Papez [46], be liable to the same pathological process(es) responsible for TGA, thus producing different variants of TGA?

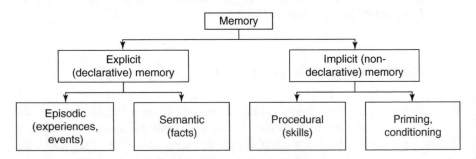

Fig. 2.2 Simplified taxonomy of memory processes (adapted from [40])

A number of potential variants of TGA have been described in the literature: transient topographical amnesia, transient partial verbal amnesia, transient semantic amnesia and transient procedural amnesia. The first two of these suggest the possible fractionation of TGA into non-verbal and verbal variants. These might legitimately be considered as forms of "selective amnesia", a specification that has been used by some authors (e.g. [47–49]). However, this terminology is probably best avoided since "selective amnesia" has passed into the vernacular to denote apparent amnesia about a particular event or events that prove convenient for the person who (apparently) cannot remember.

For clinical completeness, reports of these potential variants are included here. However, such variants, if that is indeed what they are, are either rare or extremely rare and will not be considered hereafter, since they are unlikely either to be encountered clinically or to shed any additional light on the pathogenesis of TGA.

2.3.1   Transient Topographical Amnesia (TTA)

The most frequently reported variant of the possible variants of TGA is transient topographical amnesia (TTA). A number of reports of TTA have appeared, initially single cases, all of them from Italian centres [50–53], and thereafter small series ([54], $n = 8$; [55], $n - 10$), as well as cases from countries other than Italy [54, 56–58]. TTA may be identical to, or overlap with, cases labelled as "transient topographical disorientation" [59].

Stracciari [53] described the case of a woman who experienced three isolated episodes of loss of topographical memory and postulated that this was a rare form of selective non-verbal transient amnesia. Episodes were characterised by the sudden onset of failure to find the way despite spared recognition of the environment, such as landmarks or objects, postulated to reflect transient right (non-dominant) occipitotemporal region dysfunction. Impaired recognition of landmarks may be a feature of some cases (e.g. [57, 59]).

Considering the published series of TTA, these show a female predominance (all ten cases of Stracciari et al. [55]; 6 of 8 cases of Naranjo-Fernandez et al. [54]). Episodes are brief, ranging from 5 to 40 min [55] with the average duration of 24.5 min [54], hence much shorter than in typical TGA episodes (see Sect. 2.1.4). Indeed, some attacks which have been labelled as TTA apparently last only a few seconds [57]. Patient age at time of attack ranged from 51 to 84 years in the series of Stracciari et al. [55], with an average age of 69.13 ± 8.79 years in the series of Naranjo-Fernandez et al. [54]. Recurrence of up to three episodes was noted in 3 out of 10 patients [55], with a mean number of episodes of 1.75, range 1–3 [54], although some patients have many episodes over many years [57].

That TTA may be related to TGA is suggested not only on the basis of the shared brevity of the attacks in the absence of other neurological features, but also the observation of a patient with two episodes of TGA one of which ended in a typical TTA attack [60]. Attacks may occur in patients with a history of migraine ([50], and

[55], case 9), during a migraine attack [58], and may apparently be triggered by swimming [60].

Neuropsychological evaluation in 12 patients 6–12 months after recovery from TTA showed normal performance in all tasks but lower performance compared to controls in a test of spatial (geographical) orientation, but it was not known whether this deficit predated the TTA events [61]. One patient in the series of Naranjo-Fernandez et al. [54] developed dementia 6 years after the acute episode.

No diagnostic criteria have been formulated for TTA to my knowledge. One may question whether a patient with frequent attacks labelled as TTA but associated with tonic rigidity of the left limbs and imaging findings of an angioma at the right cingulate cortex [62] should qualify. Likewise, two patients with transient topographical disorientation accompanied by visual field defects and other cognitive dysfunctions [63] are doubtful as examples of TTA if this phenomenon is pathogenetically related to TGA.

2.3.2   Transient Partial Verbal Amnesia (TPVA)

A number of case reports of patients with transient amnesia characterised by a selective impairment of verbal memory with sparing of non-verbal memory, unlike typical TGA in which both are affected, have appeared [64–67], sometimes labelled transient partial verbal amnesia (TPVA) [21].

Damasio et al. [65] described a patient with relative preservation of orientation to place and familiarity with previously known persons in the context of transient impairment of verbal memory, who subsequently retained partial memory of the event. Matias-Guiu and Codina [66] reported four patients with transient amnesia affecting verbal material, but little clinical detail was provided. Okada et al. [67] reported two patients with some degree of visual memory preservation during an attack of "TGA", with quicker recovery of non-verbal memory.

The fullest account is that of Nishiyama et al. [21]. They reported a 58-year-old man examined during an attack. When sent to the hospital because of his memory problems, manifested by repeated questioning, he was able to remember the faces of newly encountered doctors but not their names. Administered the Wechsler Memory Scale-Revised during the attack, which lasted for about 10 h, there was a discrepancy between verbal (65) and visual (113) memory indices. The delayed visual recall was normal during the attack but delayed verbal memory was severely impaired; the latter normalised by the time of re-testing 2 weeks later. The authors suggested eight points as criteria for TPVA: these were essentially the seven Hodges and Warlow 1990 criteria [14] (Table 2.1) in addition to the requirement that amnesia must be limited to verbal materials.

Yildiz et al. [68] reported a 63-year-old vasculopath who underwent coronary and lower extremity angiography who "experienced transient partial amnesia, headache, and right upper extremity numbness" after repeated injections. No other details of the neuropsychological deficit were given in the publication, but all symptoms returned to normal on the same day. Brady [69] commented on this article but added no further case. The report by Yildiz et al. [68] would not fulfil the suggested criteria for TPVA published some years earlier by Nishiyama et al. [21].

Mon et al. reported a neurologist who had a brief (<1 h; see Sect. 2.1.4) episode of amnesia during a panel consultation by video link (Zoom), confirmed as TGA by the subsequent observation of the typical magnetic resonance neuroimaging findings (Sect. 5.1.2) who "partially remembered what had happened during memory loss" [70].

The fractionation of memory function into verbal and non-verbal components might be anticipated to result in partial syndromes selectively affecting verbal memory or visual memory (TTA), perhaps reflecting selective or predominant involvement of only one cerebral hemisphere by whatever process(es) underpin(s) TGA.

2.3.3   Transient Semantic Amnesia

Hodges [71] reported a 50-year-old man who suffered an attack characterised by transient loss of memory for word and object meaning during a typical migraine headache. Interictal brain imaging (CT) and EEG were normal. This transient loss of semantic memory but with preservation of anterograde episodic and working memory was suggested to represent "transient semantic amnesia". The literature review identified only one prior possible case: Kapur et al. [72] reported a patient with temporary loss of memory for people. A report of "transient selective amnesia" for merchandise prices [47] might possibly represent a similar entity.

Considering the mental structure of memory processes, such a semantic variant of TGA might be predictable. However, to my knowledge, no subsequent similar cases have been reported, although as Hodges [71] pointed out such cases might easily be overlooked because of the more subtle cognitive dysfunction compared to that occurring in definite TGA.

2.3.4   Transient Procedural Amnesia

As previously mentioned, fractionation of memory into declarative (explicit) and non-declarative (implicit, procedural) components underlies current models of memory function (Fig. 2.2). Although all the possible variants of TGA described hitherto have involved aspects of declarative memory, it would be theoretically and clinically notable if cases of transient non-declarative memory dysfunction were also observed. Preservation of procedural memory during definite TGA cases is well attested to, including activities such as driving long distances (e.g. [73, 74]), teaching school classes [18], being interviewed for a job [75], and undertaking musical performance, either playing an instrument [76, 77] or conducting [78].

In contrast to these observations, Stracciari et al. [79] described the case of a man who experienced transient amnesia for familiar daily tasks which comprised his occupation of bread making. The authors postulated that this was a disorder similar to TGA but which selectively affected procedural memory, hence transient procedural amnesia.

To my knowledge, no subsequent cases have been reported under the rubric of transient procedural amnesia. However, Yamaoka et al. [49] reported two cases of "transient selective amnesia" lasting several hours in which the patients became unable to operate simple machines, respectively, a taxi meter and a fax machine; neither patient had evidence of anterograde amnesia. (Note that the clinical phenotype in these patients appears to differ from that in a previous case reported as "transient selective amnesia" by Finkel [47]). Moreover, both patients showed high-intensity signal lesions in the left hippocampus CA1 region on diffusion-weighted magnetic resonance imaging which disappeared in the chronic phase; such imaging changes are those typically found in TGA cases (Sect. 5.1.2). This appears to be the most compelling evidence presented to date for the existence of selective variants of TGA and might be adduced as rationale for adding neuroimaging findings to the diagnostic criteria (Sect. 2.2.2).

2.3.5   Transient Retrograde Amnesia

The term transient retrograde amnesia has been used on occasion [48, 80, 81], but whether this terminology refers to the same clinical syndrome in each instance is not clear. It has been used to describe a focal deficit in verbal fluency and living/non-living dissociation in an amnesic period following a mild head injury [81]; a syndrome of focal and selective loss of memory for autobiographical events [48]; and retrograde amnesia for recent events following anterior communicating artery aneurysm coiling ([80]; note that TGA has also been described after aneurysm coiling [82]). The duration of some of these events puts them well outside the diagnostic criteria for TGA (e.g. 10 days [81]; no improvement after 2 days [80]). On the basis of the current evidence, a selective retrograde amnesic variant of TGA is not established.

2.4   Summary and Recommendations

TGA is a relatively stereotyped syndrome of dense anterograde amnesia with variably extensive retrograde amnesia, for which clinical diagnostic criteria have been formulated and widely implemented. Whether variant forms of TGA exist, as might be predicted from the current understanding of the fractionated neuropsychological substrates of memory, remains uncertain.

Not all reports of "TGA" predating the clinical diagnostic criteria conform to what would now be considered TGA. Cases labelled as "TGA" which have been reported since the inception of these criteria but which do not apply or fulfil these criteria should be treated with some scepticism and should prompt consideration of the differential diagnosis of TGA, which is elaborated in the next chapter.

References

1. Fisher CM, Adams RD. Transient global amnesia. Trans Am Neurol Assoc. 1958;83:143–6.
2. Fisher CM, Adams RD. Transient global amnesia. Acta Neurol Scand. 1964;40(Suppl9):1–81.
3. Bender MB. Syndrome of isolated episode of confusion with amnesia. J Hillside Hosp. 1956;5:212–5.
4. Guyotat MM, Courjon J. Les ictus amnésiques. J Med Lyon. 1956;37:697–701.
5. Hainselin M, Quinette P, Desgranges B, et al. Awareness of disease state without explicit knowledge of memory failure in transient global amnesia. Cortex. 2012;48:1079–84.
6. Ahn S, Kim W, Lee YS, et al. Transient global amnesia: seven years of experience with diffusion-weighted imaging in an emergency department. Eur Neurol. 2011;65:123–8.
7. Quinette P, Guillery-Girard B, Dayan J, de la Sayette V, Marquis S, Viader F, Desgranges B, Eustache F. What does transient global amnesia really mean? Review of the literature and thorough study of 142 cases. Brain. 2006;129:1640–58.
8. Kim SH, Park YH, Kim SY, Kim JS. Impaired smooth pursuit during transient global amnesia. J Clin Neurol. 2019;15:301–7.
9. Inzitari D, Pantoni L, Lamassa M, Pallanti S, Pracucci G, Marini P. Emotional arousal and phobia in transient global amnesia. Arch Neurol. 1997;54:866–73.
10. Noël A, Quinette P, Dayan J, et al. Influence of depressive symptoms on memory in transient global amnesia. J Neuropsychol. 2017;11:108–21.
11. Noël A, Quinette P, Guillery-Girard B, et al. Psychopathological factors, memory disorders and transient global amnesia. Br J Psychiatry. 2008;193:145–51.
12. Oehler E, Iaxx F, Larre P, Ghawche F. Transient global amnesia: a descriptive study of 12 Polynesian patients [in French]. Rev Neurol (Paris). 2015;171:662–8.
13. Hoyer C, Higashida K, Fabbian F, et al. Chronobiology of transient global amnesia. J Neurol. 2022;269:361–7.
14. Hodges JR, Warlow CP. Syndromes of transient amnesia: towards a classification. A study of 153 cases. J Neurol Neurosurg Psychiatry. 1990;53:834–43.
15. Agosti C, Borroni B, Akkawi NM, Padovani A. Cerebrovascular risk factors and triggers in transient global amnesia patients with and without jugular valve incompetence: results from a sample of 243 patients. Eur Neurol. 2010;63:291–4.
16. Romoli M, Tuna MA, Li L, et al. Time trends, frequency, characteristics and prognosis of short-duration transient global amnesia. Eur J Neurol. 2020;27:887–93.
17. Lerner AJ. Diagnostic criteria in neurology. Totawa, NJ: Humana Press; 2006.
18. Kane CA. Transient global amnesia: a common, benign condition. The need for exact diagnostic criteria. West J Med. 1983;138:725–7.
19. Caplan LB. [sic]. Transient global amnesia. In: Frederiks JAM, editor. Handbook of clinical neurology. Volume 1 (45). Clinical neuropsychology. Amsterdam: Elsevier Science Publishers; 1985. p. 205–18.
20. Hodges JR. Transient amnesia. Clinical and neuropsychological aspects. London: WB Saunders; 1991.
21. Nishiyama KHK, Bandoh M, Ishikawa T, Sugishita M. Transient partial verbal amnesia. J Neurol Neurosurg Psychiatry. 1993;56:1234–5.

22. Michel P, Beaud V, Eskandari A, Maeder P, Demonet JF, Eskioglou E. Ischemic amnesia: causes and outcome. Stroke. 2017;48:2270–3.
23. Regard M, Landis T. Transient global amnesia: neuropsychological dysfunction during attack and recovery in two "pure" cases. J Neurol Neurosurg Psychiatry. 1984;47:668–72.
24. Stracciari A, Rebucci GG, Gallassi R. Transient global amnesia: neuropsychological study of a "pure" case. J Neurol. 1987;243:126–7.
25. Irioka T, Yamanami A, Yaqi Y, Mizusawa H. Aortic dissection as a possible cause of pure transient global amnesia: a case report and literature review. Neurol Sci. 2009;30:255–8.
26. Kaveeshvar H, Kashouty R, Loomba V, Yono N. A rare case of aortic dissection presenting as pure transient global amnesia. Cardiovasc J Afr. 2015;26:e8–9.
27. Michel D, Garnier P, Schneider F, Poujois A, Barral FG, Thomas-Antérion C. Diffusion MRI in pure transient global amnesia associated with bilateral vertebral artery dissection. Cerebrovasc Dis. 2004;17:264–6.
28. Beyrouti R, Mansour M, Kacem A, Zaouali J, Mrissa R. Transient global amnesia like syndrome associated with acute infarction of the corpus callosum: a case report. Acta Neurol Belg. 2016;116:375–7.
29. Fujimoto H, Imaizumi T, Nishimura Y, et al. Neurosyphilis showing transient global amnesia-like attacks and magnetic resonance imaging abnormalities mainly in the limbic system. Intern Med. 2001;40:439–42.
30. Gaul C, Dietrich W, Tomandi B, Neundörfer B, Erbguth FJ. Aortic dissection presenting with transient global amnesia-like symptoms. Neurology. 2004;63:2442–3.
31. Semmler A, Klein A, Moskau S, Linnebank M. Transient global amnesia-like episode in a patient with severe hyperhomocysteinaemia. Eur J Neurol. 2007;14:e5–6.
32. Stracciari A, Guarino M, Crespi C, Pazzaglia P. Transient amnesia triggered by acute marijuana intoxication. Eur J Neurol. 1999;6:521–3.
33. Tsai MY, Tsai MH, Yang SC, Tseng YL, Chuang YC. Transient global amnesia-like episode due to mistaken intake of zolpidem: drug safety concern in the elderly. J Patient Saf. 2009;5:32–4.
34. Carota A, Lysandropoulos AP, Calabrese P. Pure left hippocampal stroke: a transient global amnesia-plus syndrome. J Neurol. 2012;259:989–92.
35. Förster A, Griebe M, Gass A, Kern R, Hennerici MG, Szabo K. Diffusion-weighted imaging for the differential diagnosis of disorders affecting the hippocampus. Cerebrovasc Dis. 2012;33:104–15.
36. Szabo K, Hoyer C, Caplan LR, et al. Diffusion-weighted MRI in transient global amnesia and its diagnostic implications. Neurology. 2020;95:e206–12.
37. Agosti C, Borroni B, Akkawi NM, De Maria G, Padovani A. Transient global amnesia and brain lesions: new hints into clinical criteria. Eur J Neurol. 2008;15:981–4.
38. Ozkul-Wermester O, Lefaucheur R, Macaigne V, Guegan-Massardeir E, Bourre B. Transient global amnesia revealing multiple sclerosis. Presse Med. 2016;45:262–4.
39. Shanmugarajah PD, Alty J, Lily O, Ford HL. Lesson of the month 2: transient reversible amnesia in multiple sclerosis. Clin Med. 2017;17:88–90.
40. Williamson J, Larner AJ. Transient global amnesia. Br J Hosp Med. 2015;76:C186–8.
41. Caselli RJ, Tariot PN. Alzheimer's disease and its variants: a diagnostic and therapeutic guide. Oxford: Oxford University Press; 2010.
42. Dubois B, Feldman HH, Jacova C, et al. Advancing research diagnostic criteria for Alzheimer's disease: the IWG-2 criteria. Lancet Neurol. 2014;13:614–29. [Erratum Lancet Neurol. 2014;13:757]
43. Doran M, du Plessis DG, Enevoldson TP, Fletcher NA, Ghadiali E, Larner AJ. Pathological heterogeneity of clinically diagnosed corticobasal degeneration. J Neurol Sci. 2003;216:127–34.
44. Schacter DL, Tulving E. Memory systems. Cambridge: MIT Press; 1994.
45. Bennett MR, Hacker PMS. Philosophical foundations of neuroscience. Oxford: Blackwell; 2003.
46. Papez JW. A proposed mechanism of emotion. Arch Neurol Psychiatr. 1937;38:725–43. [Reprinted in J Neuropsychiatry Clin Neurosci. 1995;7:103-12.]

47. Finkel N. Transient selective amnesia for merchandise prices. Mt Sinai J Med. 1974;41:125–6.
48. McCarthy RA, Pengas G. Transient retrograde amnesia: a focal and selective (but temporary) loss of memory for autobiographical events. Cortex. 2015;64:426–8.
49. Yamaoka Y, Bandoh M, Kawai K. Reversible hippocampal lesions detected on magnetic resonance imaging in two cases of transient selective amnesia for simple machine operation. Neurocase. 2016;22:387–91.
50. Mazzoni M, Del Torto E, Vista M, Moretti P. Transient topographical amnesia: a case report. Ital J Neurol Sci. 1993;14:633–6.
51. Moretti G, Caffarra P, Manzoni GC, Scarano C, Arnone F. Transitory topographical amnesia [in Italian]. Acta Biomed Ateneo Parmense. 1981;52:119–22.
52. Moretti G, Caffarra P, Parma M. Transient topographical amnesia. Ital J Neurol Sci. 1983;4:361.
53. Stracciari A. Transient topographical amnesia. Ital J Neurol Sci. 1992;13:593–6.
54. Naranjo-Fernandez C, Arjona A, Quiroga-Subirana P, et al. Transient topographical amnesia: a description of a series of eight case [in Spanish]. Rev Neurol. 2010;50:217–20.
55. Stracciari A, Lorusso S, Pazzaglia P. Transient topographical amnesia. J Neurol Neurosurg Psychiatry. 1994;57:1423–5.
56. Pai MC, Hsiao SS. Transient partial amnesia presenting as topographical disorientation. Acta Neurol Taiwanica. 2002;11:155–7.
57. Shindo A, Satoh M, Kajikawa H, Ito N, Miyamura H, Tomimoto H. Recurrent transient topographical amnesia: a patient with frequent episodes. J Neurol. 2011;258:1566–7.
58. Yohannan DG, Watson RS, John NJ. "Lost my way"—transient topographic amnesia: a bizarre manifestation of migraine. Ann Indian Acad Neurol. 2018;21:341–3.
59. Gil-Néciga E, Alberca R, Boza F, et al. Transient topographical disorientation. Eur Neurol. 2002;48:191–9.
60. Stracciari A. Transient global amnesia and transient topographical amnesia: an observation favouring the hypothesis of a common pathogenesis. J Neurol. 2003;250:633–4.
61. Stracciari A, Lorusso S, Delli Ponti A, Mattarozzi K, Tempestini A. Cognitive functions after transient topographical amnesia. Eur J Neurol. 2002;9:401–5.
62. Cammalleri R, Gangitano M, D'Amelio M, Raieli V, Raimondo D, Camarda R. Transient topographical amnesia and cingulate cortex damage: a case report. Neuropsychologia. 1996;34:321–6.
63. Ajmard G, Vighetto A, Confavreaux C, Devic M. La desorientation spatiale. Rev Neurol (Paris). 1981;137:97–111.
64. Berthier ML, Starkstein SE. Transient partial amnesia. J Neuropsychiatry Clin Neurosci. 1990;2:465–6.
65. Damasio AR, Graff-Radford NR, Damasio H. Transient partial amnesia. Arch Neurol. 1983;40:656–7.
66. Matias-Guiu J, Codina A. Transient global amnesia: criteria and classification [letter]. Neurology. 1986;36:441–2.
67. Okada F, Ito N, Tsukamoto R. Two cases of transient partial amnesia in the course of transient global amnesia. J Clin Psychiatry. 1987;48:449–50.
68. Yildiz A, Yencilek E, Apaydin FD, Duce MN, Ozer C, Atalay A. Transient partial amnesia complicating cardiac and peripheral arteriography with nonionic contrast medium. Eur Radiol. 2003;13(Suppl4):L113–5.
69. Brady AP. Transient partial amnesia following coronary and peripheral arteriography. Eur Radiol. 2005;15:1493–4.
70. Mon Y, Isono O, Takaoka S, Tokura N. A neurologist who suffered from transient global/partial amnesia: a case report. eNeurologica Sci. 2021;24:100347.
71. Hodges JR. Transient semantic amnesia: a new syndrome? J Neurol Neurosurg Psychiatry. 1997;63:548–9.
72. Kapur N, Katifi H, El-Zawawi H, Sedgewick M, Barker S. Transient memory loss for people. J Neurol Neurosurg Psychiatry. 1994;57:862–4.

73. Gordon B, Marin O. Transient global amnesia: an extensive case report. J Neurol Neurosurg Psychiatry. 1979;42:572–5.
74. Huang CF, Pai MC. Transient amnesia in a patient with left temporal tumor. Symptomatic transient global amnesia or an epileptic amnesia? Neurologist. 2008;14:196–200.
75. Caplan L, Chedru F, Lhermitte F, Mayman C. Transient global amnesia and migraine. Neurology. 1981;31:1167–70.
76. Byer JA, Crowley WJ Jr. Musical performance during transient global amnesia. Neurology. 1980;30:80–2.
77. Thakur K, Ropper A. Transient global amnesia during a professional cello concert. J Clin Neurosci. 2011;18:1260–1.
78. Evers S, Frese A, Bethke F. Conducting without memory—a case report on transient global amnesia. Eur J Neurol. 2002;9:695–6.
79. Stracciari A, Guarino M, Pazzaglia P. Transient procedural amnesia. Ital J Neurol Sci. 1997;18:35–6.
80. Kamble RB, Sheshadri V, Jayaraman A, Chandramouli BA. Rare complication of anterior communicating artery coiling: transient retrograde amnesia. Neuroradiol J. 2015;28:325–8.
81. Papagno C. Transient retrograde amnesia associated with impaired naming of living categories. Cortex. 1998;34:111–21.
82. Graff-Radford J, Clapp AJ, Lanzino G, Rabinstein AA. Transient amnesia after coiling of a posterior circulation aneurysm. Neurocrit Care. 2013;18:245–7.

Chapter 3
Differential Diagnosis of TGA

Abstract This chapter considers the differential diagnosis of TGA. Key considerations include cerebrovascular disease (TIA, stroke), epilepsy (transient epileptic amnesia, TEA) and psychological causes, as well as a variety of other causes of transient amnesia (migraine, adverse drug effect, hypoglycaemia, head injury) and transient cerebral disorder (delirium, infection). On clinical grounds alone, it is often possible to distinguish TGA from other causes of transient amnesia.

Keywords TGA · TEA · TIA · Psychogenic amnesia

There are a number of symptomatic causes of amnesia [1, 2] which, if transient (Table 3.1), may sometimes be mistaken for TGA. However, the differential diagnosis of TGA covers more than just amnesic syndromes (Table 3.2). Some of these conditions will be considered in this chapter.

As may be expected for an acute and transient syndrome, most patients with transient global amnesia (TGA) who come to medical attention are seen by primary care physicians working in community settings or acute care physicians based in district general hospitals rather than by cognitive neurologists in dedicated tertiary neuroscience centres (unless specific services and care pathways have been established). In one small survey involving eight definite cases seen by one neurologist, three were seen in outpatient clinics, five as ward consultations; the majority (7/8, = 88%) were seen in district general hospitals. Of note, the working or suggested diagnoses (sometimes more than one) of the referring clinicians, which were available in seven cases at the time of referral to the neurologist, were stroke or TIA (5 cases), epilepsy (2) and viral illness (1) [4]. Certainly, the former two diagnoses feature prominently in the differential diagnosis of TGA, which also encompasses psychiatric or psychological disorder ([5], p.49–57).

The contrasts between TGA and some of these other conditions are summarised in Table 3.3, although this should not be taken to imply that the clinical differences are always necessarily clear cut. The differential diagnosis of TGA is considered here in greater detail.

© The Author(s), under exclusive license to Springer Nature
Switzerland AG 2022
A.J. Larner, *Transient Global Amnesia*,
https://doi.org/10.1007/978-3-030-98939-2_3

Table 3.1: Differential diagnosis of amnesia (adapted from [3], p.242–3)

- Acute/transient:
  Transient global amnesia (TGA)
  Transient epileptic amnesia (TEA)
  Transient psychological amnesia (TPA)
  Migraine
  Adverse drug effect
  Hypoglycaemia
  Traumatic brain (closed head) injury
- Chronic/persistent:
  Alzheimer's disease
  Wernicke–Korsakoff syndrome
  Sequela of herpes simplex encephalitis
  Limbic encephalitis (paraneoplastic or non-paraneoplastic)
  Hypoxic brain injury
  Bilateral paramedian thalamic infarction/posterior cerebral artery occlusion ("strategic infarct dementia")
  Third ventricle tumour, cyst; fornix damage
  Temporal lobectomy (bilateral, or unilateral with previous contralateral injury, usually birth asphyxia)
  Focal retrograde amnesia

Table 3.2: Differential diagnosis of TGA

- Causes of transient amnesia:
  Transient epileptic amnesia (TEA)
  Transient psychological amnesia (TPA)
  Migraine
  Adverse drug effect
  Hypoglycaemia
  Traumatic brain (closed head) injury
  Alcohol-induced amnesia
  Fatigue amnesia
- Causes of acute cerebral disorder:
  Transient ischaemic attack (TIA)
  Acute confusional state/delirium/toxic-metabolic encephalopathy
  Intracerebral haemorrhage/subarachnoid haemorrhage
  Acute brain infection (encephalitis)

3.1 Cerebrovascular Disease

In the light of the apparently sudden onset of neurological dysfunction in TGA, it is easy to understand why the possibility of cerebrovascular disease featured amongst the pathogenic considerations in early descriptions of the disorder, such as those of Guyotat and Courjon (1956) [7], Poser and Ziegler (1960) [8] and Halsey (1967) [9]. Fisher and Adams noted in their monograph on TGA that "[t]he possibility that such an episode might have been the first evidence of an approaching stroke … was responsible for our seeing so many of these patients" ([10], p.46). Clinicians unfamiliar with TGA may still consider stroke or transient ischaemic attack (TIA) as

Table 3.3: Comparison of typical features of transient global amnesia (TGA), transient epileptic amnesia (TEA), transient ischaemic attack (TIA) and transient psychological amnesia (TPA) (adapted from [6])

Clinical feature	TGA	TEA	TIA	TPA
Anterograde amnesia during attack	Yes	Yes	Yes	No
Focal neurological deficits	No	No	Yes	No
Aura, automatisms	No	Yes	No	No
Symptom duration	<24 h	Usually <1 h	<24 h	Variable
Recurrence rate	Low	High	Varied	Varied
Triggers	Emotional stress or physical exertion	Can occur on waking	No	Emotional stress
Responds to antiepileptic drugs	No	Yes	No	No
EEG abnormalities during attack	No	Yes	No	No

foremost amongst the possible causes [4], justifiably since stroke was the most important differential diagnosis of in a recent large series of suspected TGA cases (6.6%) [11].

On occasion, TGA has been associated with various cerebrovascular events, including infarction and haemorrhage, both arterial and venous, TIA and other conditions affecting the vasculature. Some of these reports have involved memory eloquent brain substrates (medial temporal lobe, thalamus, fornix, corpus callosum, hippocampus), elements within the circuit described by Papez [12], and hence plausible as causes of memory disorder. However, caveats apply before a causal relation between these cerebrovascular disorders and TGA may be accepted. For example (as previously mentioned, see Sect. 2.2.1), many of these cases were reported prior to the definition of widely accepted diagnostic criteria for TGA, and the presence of possible confounding factors may sometimes be identified. Cases of posterior circulation stroke or TIA and of TGA may be elided in some reports. For example, at least one of Lou's (1968) patients with "repeated TGA" probably had ischaemic events (3 episodes causing a persistent memory deficit which gradually improved, along with a right upper quadrantanopia and right limb paraesthesia) [13]. Likewise, de Tribolet et al. [14] reported six cases of cortical blindness and amnesia, which were likely to be due to stroke, but also two cases of transient "Korsakoff's syndrome", more likely to have been examples of TGA. Posterior cerebral artery occlusion is a recognised cause of amnesia (e.g. [15]), and transient amnesia has been reported on occasion to herald brainstem infarction (e.g. [16, 17]). A TGA-like syndrome ("TGA plus") has been reported in pure hippocampal stroke with additional aphasia [18] and in corpus callosum infarction [19], although the nosological position of "TGA-like syndrome" is questionable (Sect. 2.2.2). These entities might be better labelled "amnesic stroke". Certainly amnesia, both persistent and transient, can be a result of strategic infarcts (e.g. [20, 21]).

With the advent of magnetic resonance (MR) brain imaging, the frequent observation of focal punctate areas of high signal change in the hippocampus on diffusion-weighted imaging MR sequences (MR-DWI) has been interpreted as evidence of cerebral ischaemia, albeit not typical of infarction (see Sect. 5.1.2, especially Sect. 5.1.2.6 for a discussion of the pathogenesis of these imaging changes).

3.1.1 Transient Ischaemic Attack (TIA)

Arguments against TGA being a form of TIA include both clinical and epidemiological considerations. TIAs are usually accompanied by focal neurological signs (e.g. hemiparesis, amaurosis fugax) which are absent from TGA (by definition, according to the 1990 diagnostic criteria of Hodges and Warlow [22]; see Sect. 2.2.2 and Table 2.1). Furthermore, episodes of TGA are usually isolated, whereas recurrence rates are much higher in TIA (Table 3.3), sometimes with progression to established stroke, which is not seen in TGA. Comparison of vascular risk factors in patients with TGA and TIA has generally found a significantly greater prevalence in the latter group, with the risk factor profile in TGA patients resembling that of normal controls (see Sect. 7.11 for extended discussion).

Chen et al. [23] described a patient (M76) with "a spell of TGA" followed by several episodes of amaurosis fugax (ocular TIA) who was found on investigation to have progressive occlusion of the right common carotid artery. The concurrence of events was taken to imply a vascular aetiology for TGA.

3.1.2 Stroke: Cerebral Infarction

Occasional cases with the typical clinical phenotype of TGA and with computed tomography (CT) changes indicative of established ischaemic stroke were reported when this neuroimaging modality first became widely available (e.g. [24–26]).

With the advent of higher resolution magnetic resonance imaging (MRI), further cases were identified. A narrative review [27] (Table 3.4) found descriptions of TGA in association with infarction in various locations, including the medial temporal lobe [28–32], hippocampus [18, 31, 33–40], fornix [41, 42], thalamus [43–45], cingulate gyrus or bundle [46–48], striatum (caudate and putamen) [49–53], corpus callosum [19, 54] and frontal lobe [39, 55]. Thus, these strokes involved memory eloquent brain structures, linked through Papez circuit [12], in many cases, as well as frontal lobe structures involved in the organisation and monitoring of memory processes, but with an absence of significant hemisphere strokes. This localisation suggests that stroke-related TGA might be regarded as a (rare) symptomatic (or secondary) form of TGA. Possible pathogenic reasons for the occasional concurrence of ischaemic stroke and TGA are considered later (Sect. 9.2.1). Suffice it to say here that the phenotype of TGA may occur on rare occasions in association with established stroke on neuroimaging.

Table 3.4: Reports of MR-confirmed acute infarction or stroke associated with the clinical phenotype of TGA

Location	Reference	Demographic and other clinical features	MR imaging findings
Temporal lobe			
	Greer et al. (2001) [28]	F77	Left mesial temporal lobe ischaemic infarct
	López-Pesquera et al. (2005) [29]	F49	Tiny ischaemic stroke in white matter of left temporal lobe
	Graff-Radford et al. (2013) [30]	F56; following coiling of small posterior circulation cerebral aneurysm	Small medial temporal lobe strokes
	Duan et al. (2016) [31]	M72; coronary angiography	Acute infarction in left hippocampus and temporal lobe
	Ramanathan & Wachsman (2021) [32] ($n = 2$)	F48 history of hypertension, COVID-19 +ve F71 history of hypertension, COVID-19 +ve	Bilateral medial temporal lobe infarcts Small R temporal lobe infarct
Hippocampus			
	Adler et al. (2012) [33]	F65	Subtle ischaemic region in the right hippocampus compatible with acute infarct
	Carota et al. (2012) [18]	R41; "TGA plus" (anomic pauses, "amnesic aphasia"); patent foramen ovale	Acute infarct, dorsal part of left hippocampal body
	Gungor-Tuncer et al. (2012) [34] and (2015) [35] (case 2)	F62; history of migraine	Left pons (7h); left hippocampal and right frontal areas (36h)
	Li and Hu (2013) [36]	M61	Bilateral hippocampal lesions, acute ischaemia
	Gungor-Tuncer et al. (2015) [35] (case 1)	F56; history of migraine	Two punctate acute infarcts in the left hippocampus
	Duan et al. (2016) [31] ($n = 2$)	M73; cerebral angiography, vertebral artery angioplasty M72; coronary angiography	Acute infarction in left hippocampus Acute infarction in left hippocampus and temporal lobe
	Naldi et al. (2017) [37]	F82	Right posterior hippocampal stroke
	Yun et al. (2017) [38]	M68	Bilateral hippocampal lesions

(continued)

Table 3.4: (continued)

Location	Reference	Demographic and other clinical features	MR imaging findings
	Kang et al. (2021) [39]	M54	Right frontal and hippocampus strokes
	Sakihara et al. (2021) [40]	F35; septic embolus from infective endocarditis	Right hippocampus
Fornix			
	Gupta et al. (2015) [41]	F66; paroxysmal atrial fibrillation	Body and left column of fornix infarction
	Meyer (2016) [42]	N/A	Left fornix infarction
Thalamus			
	Pradalier et al. (2000) [43]	F54; history of migraine without aura	Right anteroinferior thalamic ischaemic lesion
	Giannantoni et al. (2015) [44]	F69	Thalamic ischaemic lesion
	Dogan et al. (2017) [45]	F65	Left thalamus and left paramedian mesencephalon infarcts
Cingulate gyrus			
	Gallardo-Tur et al. (2014) [46]	M62; two TGA episodes	Acute ischaemic stroke of small size (15 mm maximal diameter) at right cingulate gyrus
	Chau and Liu (2019) [47]	F60	Left cingulate gyrus
	Meng et al. (2021) [48]	F89; history of hypertension	L retrosplenial infarct (cingulate bundle and retrosplenial cortex)
Striatum (caudate, putamen)			
	Ravindran et al. (2004) [49]	M56	Acute ischaemia in the body of right caudate nucleus
	Kim et al. (2012) [50]	F63	L putamen acute microinfarct
	Koltermann et al. (2015) [51]	M50	Acute ischaemic lacunar infarction, head of caudate nucleus
	Yoshida (2017) [52]	F67	Lacunar infarction of the left putamen
	Tarazona et al. (2021) [53]	F89; history of migraine	R lenticular nucleus (outermost putamen)
Corpus callosum			
	Saito et al. (2003) [54]	M58	Small lesion of high signal intensity in the left retrosplenium of the corpus callosum

(continued)

Table 3.4: (continued)

Location	Reference	Demographic and other clinical features	MR imaging findings
	Beyrouti et al. (2016) [19]	M62	Infarction of genu and body of corpus callosum
Frontal lobe			
	Kim et al. (2018) [55] (*n* – 3)	No details	1. Left orbitofrontal. 2. Left prefrontal. 3. Right frontal and left parietal.
	Kang et al. (2021) [39]	M54	Right frontal and hippocampus strokes

Table 3.5: Reports of cerebral haemorrhage or haematoma associated with the clinical phenotype of TGA

	Location	Reference(s)
Haemorrhage		
	Left temporal haemorrhage	Landi et al. 1982 [60]
	Subarachnoid haemorrhage	Sandyk 1984 [63] Monzani et al. 2000 [61]
	Left frontal haemorrhage	Jacome and Yanez 1988 [59]
	Haemorrhage into a tumour	Sorenson et al. 1995 [64] Honma and Nagao 1996 [58]
	Cingulate gyrus haemorrhage	Yoon et al. 2006 [65]
Haematoma		
	Intraventricular haematoma	Heon et al. 1972 [57]
	Subdural haematoma	Chatham and Brillman 1985 [56]
	Left thalamic haematoma	Moonis et al. 1988 [62]

3.1.3   Stroke: Cerebral Haemorrhage

Intracranial haemorrhage (intracerebral, subdural or subarachnoid) may potentially be confused with TGA by virtue of its acute onset, but amnesia is seldom a prominent feature, and there is often impairment of consciousness. Intracranial haemorrhage or haematoma has on occasion been reported in association with TGA [56–65] (see Table 3.5), but the exact diagnostic status of such cases is uncertain, possibilities including misdiagnosis of TGA or chance concurrence.

3.1.4   Cerebral Vasculopathies

TGA has been reported on occasion with a variety of other disorders affecting the cerebral vasculature.

An amnesic syndrome following anterior communicating artery rupture and/or surgery is well recognised, but only one account of cerebral aneurysm associated with transient amnesia resembling TGA has been found. The event was apparently triggered by a coiling procedure in the posterior circulation, with evidence of medial temporal lobe strokes found on diffusion-weighted MR imaging [30].

Intracranial dural arteriovenous fistula (dAVF) may sometimes present with cognitive deficits suggestive of a dementia syndrome (e.g. [66]), sometimes rapidly progressing [67]. However, only two definite reports of TGA with dAVF have been identified [68, 69], one with recurrent events [68]. The patient reported by Heine et al. [70] might be another example (see [71], p.189).

Occasional cases of TGA have been reported in association with the reversible cerebral vasoconstriction syndrome (RCVS), a condition typically characterised by severe headaches, including thunderclap headache, and reversible segmental cerebral artery vasoconstriction which may be complicated by ischaemic or haemorrhagic stroke [72–74]. Like migraine (Sect. 3.4.1 and Sect. 7.9) and primary headache associated with sexual activity (Sect. 8.4), headache in this context may be a consequence of activation of the trigeminocervical complex. The posterior reversible encephalopathy syndrome (PRES) may be related to RCVS, sharing some features and risk factors. PRES is typically characterised by headache, visual field and motor deficits, confusion, impaired consciousness and seizures, again with ischaemic or haemorrhagic lesions. TGA has on occasion been described in association with PRES [75, 76].

Other disorders sometimes associated with vasculopathy that have on occasion been reported in association with TGA include Sneddon syndrome [77], scleroderma [78] and cerebral autosomal dominant arteriopathy with subcortical infarcts and leukoencephalopathy (CADASIL) [79].

Thrombotic tendencies might be relevant to TGA pathogenesis, secondary to cerebral venous outflow obstruction, as, for example, in antiphospholipid antibody syndrome in which TGA has occasionally been reported ([80, 81]; possibly [82]). However, venous thrombosis of cerebral [83, 84] or cervical (jugular) veins [85] has rarely been reported in association with TGA (see Sect. 9.2.2 for discussion of venous outflow obstruction as a possible aetiological factor in some cases of TGA).

3.1.5   Cerebral Angiography

One of the earliest possible reports of TGA (see Sect. 1.2) related to catheter angiography of the vertebral artery [86]. Further instances of angiography-related memory disturbance, some of which may be cases of TGA, have been reported (Table 3.6), involving procedures visualising both cerebral (carotid or vertebral) and coronary arterial vasculature (but apparently not peripheral limb vasculature [31]). One case related to renal artery angiography has been reported [124]. The procedural use of benzodiazepines (Sect. 3.4.2) may be a confounding factor in some of these reports.

The mechanism(s) by which angiography might trigger TGA remain(s) uncertain. Suggestions have included arterial spasm and the injection of contrast material (both ionic and non-ionic). Neuroradiological evidence of ischaemia, in the form of

Table 3.6: Reports of angiography and dissection associated with the clinical phenotype of TGA

		References
Angiography	Cerebral	Hauge (1954) ($n = 3$) [86]
		Deak and Toth (1964) [87]
		Whishart 1971 [88]
		de Tribolet et al. (1975) [14]
		Wales and Nov (1981) ($n = 2$) [89]
		Cochran et al. (1982) ($n = 7$) [90]
		Haas (1983) [91]
		Pexman and Coates (1983) ($n = 12$) [92]
		Giang and Kido (1989) ($n = 2$) [93]
		Minuk et al. (1990) [94]
		Juni et al. (1992) [95]
		Brady et al. (1993) [96]
		Schamschula and Soo (1994) ($n = 2$) [97]
		Jackson et al. (1995) ($n = 6$) [98]
		Meder et al. (1997) [99]
		Woolfenden et al. (1997) [100]
		Kapur et al. (1998) [101]
		Tanabe et al. (1999) [102]
		Kim et al. (2006) [103]
		Foss-Skiftesvik et al. (2015) [104]
		Duan et al. (2016) ($n = 5$) [31]
		Tiu et al. (2016) [105]
		Lee (2020) [106]
	Coronary	Fischer-Williams et al. (1970) [107]
		Shuttleworth and Wise (1973) ($n = 2$) [108]
		Lockwood et al. (1983) [109]
		Koehler et al. (1986) [110]
		Yildiz et al (2003) [111]
		Kurokawa et al. (2004) ($n = 2$) [112]
		Fernandez et al. (2005) [113]
		Wong et al. 2005 [114]
		Udyavar et al. (2006) [115]
		Duan et al. (2016) ($n = 4$) [31]
Dissection	Aorta	Rosenberg (1979) [116]
		Gaul et al. (2004) [117]
		Mondon et al. (2007) [118]
		Irioka et al. (2009) [119]
		Colotto et al. (2011) [120]
		Kaveeshvar et al. (2015) [121]
	Vertebral artery	Michel et al. (2004) [122]
		Yokota et al. (2015) [123]

small acute infarctions in the hippocampus, has been documented in some cases
(e.g. [31]). Angiography-related TGA might also conceivably be related to inadvertent, iatrogenic, arterial dissection at the time of the procedure, predisposing to
embolisation. Similar explanations might pertain in a case following carotid artery
stenting followed by carotid angiography [106]). TGA has also been reported after
vertebral artery angioplasty and stenting [103].

TGA has been described with arterial dissections, of either the aorta or the verte-bral artery (Table 3.6). However, no reports of TGA in fibromuscular dysplasia, a disorder associated with arterial dissection, have been identified.

Another pathogenic possibility relates to migraine (Sect. 3.4.1 and 7.9): cer-tainly, migrainous phenomena may on occasion be triggered by angiographic pro-cedures (e.g. [125]), and this may have played a role in the angiography-related case of Fernandez et al. [113].

3.1.6   Cardiac Disorders

In addition to episodes related to coronary angiography (see Sect. 3.1.5; Table 3.6), TGA has also been reported on occasion in association with a variety of coronary syndromes including acute myocardial infarction [126–129], cardiac arrhythmia [130] and cyanotic heart disease [131]; mitral valve prolapse has also been men-tioned [132]. However, the paucity of reports suggests that these might be simply examples of chance concurrence, unrelated to the cardiac event or disorder, although cerebral hypoperfusion or embolism might occur in these situations and be a pre-cipitating factor for TGA.

A cardiac condition that might be pathogenically relevant to TGA is Takotsubo cardiomyopathy, or the "broken-heart syndrome", concurrence with which has been reported on several occasions (e.g. [133–142]). Petrea et al. speculated that the cat-echolamine surge associated with myocardial stunning in Takotsubo cardiomyopa-thy might also be associated with "cortical stunning" and hence that these conditions might have a shared pathogenesis [137]. Of possible interest, in a review of over 1100 reports of Takotsubo cardiomyopathy, emotional and physical stressors pre-ceded the syndrome in 39% and 35% of patients, respectively [143]; these are also significant recognised precipitating factors for TGA (see Sect. 8.1 and 8.2). Hence, the two conditions may have a shared pathogenesis, leading some to characterise TGA as "the cerebral Takotsubo" [144]. Myocardial injury, assessed by means of highly sensitive assays for cardiac troponin, was found in 28 of a series of 113 TGA patients [145]. It might be of interest to investigate whether the unique signature of microRNAs which has been reported to distinguish Takotsubo cardiomyopathy from acute myocardial infarction [146] is also seen in TGA.

Klötzsch et al. [147] reported an increased frequency of patent foramen ovale (PFO) in patients with TGA but this finding has not, to my knowledge, been repli-cated. PFO may be associated with paradoxical embolism, which might conceiv-ably be of relevance to TGA pathogenesis. TGA occurring immediately after right-left shunt of saline contrast during transoesophageal echocardiography has been reported [148]. Maalikjy Akkawi et al. [149] examined TGA, TIA and control patients for evidence of PFO with contrast transcranial duplex sonography but found no difference between the three groups. Noh and Kang reported that TGA patients with PFO had fewer vascular risk factors than those without PFO and suggested that paradoxical embolus might be a cause of TGA in these patients [150].

PFO is certainly associated with an increased risk of decompression sickness in divers. TGA has been reported in divers and ascribed to breathing hyperoxic mixtures, but no data on PFO were presented [151]. Cold water immersion (see Sect. 8.3) might also be relevant to diving-related TGA cases. In the light of the putative link between TGA and migraine (Sect. 7.9), the observation that PFO is probably more prevalent in patients with migraine might be significant, although whether the relationship between migraine and PFO is causal or coincident remains unclear [152].

3.2 Epilepsy

The sudden onset of neurological dysfunction in TGA has suggested to some authors the possibility of an epileptic aetiology. Fisher and Adams ([10], p.46) certainly considered it as a cause, and the possibility has recurred from time to time (e.g. [153–157]) and may still be questioned by some clinicians who are not familiar with TGA [4]. Certainly, Miller Fisher [158], a clinician with a deep knowledge of cerebrovascular disease [159–162], continued to argue that TGA was a form of seizure affecting the hippocampal-diencephalic system.

3.2.1 Transient Epileptic Amnesia (TEA)

Probably, the earliest account of attacks of transient amnesia of epileptic origin was by John Hughlings Jackson (1835–1911) in his 1888 report of his physician patient known as "Dr Z" [163]. However, although occasional cases of epileptic amnesia have subsequently been reported (e.g. [164–169]), it was not until the 1990s that the syndrome of transient epileptic amnesia (TEA) was more fully characterised by Kapur [170] and by Zeman et al. [171] and systematic studies and reviews subsequently undertaken (e.g. [172–180]). Diagnostic criteria for TEA have been suggested ([171] and [180], p.143) (Table 3.7; compare with Table 2.1).

Transient epileptic amnesia (TEA) is a distinctive epilepsy syndrome (Table 3.3), characterised by brief amnesic episodes, usually lasting 1 hour or less in duration, and often occurring on waking from sleep (Case Study 3.1). Attacks may be accompanied by other features suggestive of epilepsy such as automatisms or olfactory hallucinations. Hence, it may be worth asking patients who complain of autobiographical amnesia whether or not they also have automatisms or olfactory hallucinations as possible pointers to an epileptic aetiology. There is a high recurrence rate for episodes of TEA, contrary to the observations in TGA (Sect. 2.1.5).

Table 3.7: Diagnostic criteria for TEA (based on [171] and [180], p.143)

Recurrent witnessed episodes of transient amnesia.
Other cognitive functions intact.
Evidence of epilepsy:
(a) Other clinical features of epilepsy.
(b) Response to anticonvulsant medication.
(c) Epileptiform abnormalities on EEG.

Case Study 3.1: Transient Epileptic Amnesia (TEA)

A 43-year-old man and his wife reported episodes over 1 year in which he could not remember things on waking in the mornings, accompanied by a blank facial expression. There was also a history of accelerated forgetting of events which had occurred a couple of weeks earlier, such that he could not recall a recent holiday or conversations. The history was thought to be typical for the diagnosis of transient epileptic amnesia (TEA). The patient was unimpaired on cognitive screening instruments (Addenbrooke's Cognitive Examination-Revised score = 100/100). MR brain imaging, standard and sleep-deprived EEG were all within normal limits. Initiation of antiepileptic drug therapy (carbamazepine) was followed by a remission of episodes over a 2-year period of follow-up.

Many TEA patients also report interictal memory problems, characterised as accelerated long-term forgetting and autobiographical amnesia; the latter may be prominent [181, 182]. An accelerated loss of new information and impaired remote autobiographical memory has been demonstrated in TEA patients, but the aetiology of these deficits remains uncertain, possibilities including ongoing seizure activity, seizure-induced medial temporal lobe damage or subtle ischaemic pathology [182]. Accelerated forgetting has also been described in medial temporal lobe epilepsy [183]. Symptoms of emotional lability, in particular pathological tearfulness or labile crying in response to relatively minor stimuli, has also been reported in the context of TEA [173, 184].

The syndrome of "isolated autobiographical amnesia" [185] may be related to TEA. Likewise, some patients who have been reported with the syndrome of focal (isolated) retrograde amnesia [186] (Sect. 3.3) may have an underlying epileptic disorder, possibly related to other brain insults such as encephalitis or alcohol misuse ([187, 188]; see also discussion in [189]).

Electroencephalography (EEG) in TEA may be associated with clear-cut seizure activity during amnesic episodes. Abnormalities may be found in interictal EEG recordings in about one-third of TEA patients, although sometimes sleep-deprived EEG may be required. Magnetic resonance brain imaging may show hippocampal atrophy [190] or amygdala enlargement [191–193] (Case Study 3.2).

Management of TEA may require antiepileptic drug therapy. TEA generally responds favourably to standard antiepileptic medications such as sodium valproate, carbamazepine, lamotrigine or levetiracetam. Advice on appropriate lifestyle modifications, including reference to statutory restrictions on driving, is also an integral aspect of management.

TEA is an infrequent condition. Over the 20-year period 2002–2021 inclusive, the author has encountered only six definite cases (e.g. Case Studies 3.1 and 3.2; [192, 194]), all male, as compared to the predominance of females in cases of TGA ($n = 50$) seen over the same period (F:M = 29:21; Figure 7.2). In addition, one further possible case has been seen, in which the episodes were initially diagnosed by another consultant neurologist as parasomnias. These episodes on waking occurred at approximately the same age at onset as a more pervasive memory problem which evolved into Alzheimer's disease (AD) [195]. Epileptic seizures in AD may take a number of forms and become more frequent with disease duration although they may occur at onset of cognitive decline [196], so this concurrence might possibly reflect shared pathogenic processes involving synaptic network pathology in the medial temporal lobes [197–200]. TEA has also been suggested as a cause of wandering behaviours observed in AD patients [201].

TEA is usually idiopathic but may sometimes be secondary or symptomatic. Cases associated with medial temporal lobe mass lesions are described, some of which have also manifested episodes more typical of TGA, e.g. of longer duration, and following physical exertion [191, 192, 194, 202], prompting the suggestion that all cases of TGA associated with focal medial temporal lobe tumours are in fact TEA masquerading as TGA [194]. TEA may also on occasion be associated with neurodegenerative disease, such as AD [195, 201]. TEA has also been described as the presenting feature of autoimmune limbic encephalitis in association with various autoantibodies, including NMDAR [203], CASPR2 [204] and GABA$_B$ [205].

Whereas a family history of TGA may sometimes be uncovered (Sect. 7.8), I am aware of only two reports of a possible family history of TEA, one affecting three siblings [206], the other in a 20-year-old man, his mother and grandmother [207].

TEA enters the differential diagnosis of TGA, which it may resemble, but from which it usually differs in a number of respects, including the timing and frequency of attacks (Table 3.3). The key points of differentiation are that TEA attacks are generally briefer in duration and have a higher recurrence rate than TGA. As a rule of thumb, a cut-off of about 2 hours has been used to differentiate TEA from TGA, but some caution is needed as brief (<1 h) episodes of TGA are recognised [208]. There may also be an impression that the anterograde amnesia is denser in TGA than in TEA, patients with the latter condition having partial recall.

The "absence of epileptic features" is one of the proposed diagnostic criteria for TGA [22], although EEG is seldom performed during an episode of TGA, other than fortuitously, and is normal (e.g. [209]; Sect. 4.2.1 and 4.2.2).

3.2.2   TGA and TEA: Is there an Interrelation?

The distinction between TGA and TEA is not always as clear cut as might be implied by presentations such as Table 3.3. For example, some patients reported in the literature as having "TGA" may, in retrospect, have in fact had TEA, e.g. Greene and Bennett's patient who had amnesia on awakening and EEG abnormality [210], although Daniel ([71], p.63) seems to accept this as a case of TGA. In the Oxford TGA study, an unexpected finding was that 8 of 114 patients with apparent TGA (7%) subsequently developed epilepsy, usually of complex partial type, prompting the view that the original attacks were in fact due to seizures ([5], p.41,46–7,56,121,123,124–5,137). In a series of 64 TGA patients reported by Zorzon et al., three were eventually considered to have an epileptic aetiology [211].

Aside from diagnostic confusion, it is possible that there may be an interrelationship between TGA and TEA. Occasional patients have been reported with episodes resembling both TGA and TEA, the latter following the former, with associated medial lobe structural abnormalities on MR imaging (e.g. [191, 192, 194, 202, 212, 213]; Case Study 3.2). These cases raise the possibility that TEA and TGA are not mutually exclusive conditions but may in some instances be interrelated. In the light of the known vulnerability of hippocampal CA1 neurones to transient ischaemia (e.g. [214]) with subsequent apoptosis, perhaps TGA episodes, particularly if recurrent, might damage the hippocampus ([215, 216]; see Sect. 5.1.2 and 5.2.1) in such a way (ischaemic scarring) that the threshold for epileptic attacks is subsequently reduced (Case Study 3.2). Hence, rather than epilepsy being simply mistaken for TGA ([5], p.56), it might be that some of these cases represent an evolution from episodes of TGA to epilepsy.

Case Study 3.2: A relationship between TGA and TEA

A 66-year-old man reported four episodes of transient amnesia over a 6-month period. Each episode occurred within hours of strenuous physical exercise. In the first, he returned home from a bicycle ride confused about the route he had taken. The second event occurred following a walk up a steep incline. The third event occurred the day after a strenuous bicycle ride when the patient awoke in the morning confused as to where he was and what the plan for the day was. This confusion recurred the same day following a post-prandial nap. All the events were witnessed by the patient's wife who noted repetitive questioning to be a feature in each. All lasted between 30 min and 2 h with complete recovery. No other accompanying focal neurological symptoms were noted during the attacks.

At initial neurological assessment, neurological examination and cognitive screening were normal. The first two events were thought to be typical of exercise-related TGA, whereas the latter two had clinical features more suggestive of TEA, particularly the relationship to waking from sleep.

On further follow-up, more events occurred, exclusively related to waking from sleep. Standard electroencephalogram (EEG) was within normal limits, but sleep-deprived EEG showed excess slow waves over the right temporal region and one prolonged run of slow waves followed by brief high amplitude sharp wave bursts. Magnetic resonance (MR) brain imaging showed subtle but unequivocal enlargement of the right amygdala with normal diffusion-weighted imaging and no disruption of limbic white matter tracts or adjacent temporal fibre bundles. The patient was treated with levetiracetam (500 mg bd).

Clinical and neuroradiological follow-up of this patient now extends to 8 years. There has been complete cessation of all amnesic events since prescription of levetiracetam, with no dosage increase required. The patient has noted blank areas in his memory for distant significant personal events, suggestive of autobiographical amnesia, but cognitive screening has remained normal. MR brain imaging, initially performed annually, showed no change in the amygdala enlargement, but between year 6 and year 8 the appearances reverted to normal.

Although it is possible that all the events were epileptic in origin, another possibility is that initial attacks of TGA left residual hippocampal damage resulting in seizure activity or lowered seizure threshold [192, 194].

3.3   Transient Psychological Amnesia (TPA)

Transient amnesia of psychological origin (TPA) enters the differential diagnosis of TGA (Table 3.3). TPA has variously been designated, for example, as hysterical amnesia, fugue state, psychogenic amnesia, functional amnesia, focal retrograde amnesia and dissociative amnesia [186, 217–220].

Once thought to be common, the number of reported cases appears to have declined since the 1950s, at roughly the same time as TGA was becoming recognised as a clinical entity. It has been speculated that earlier cases of TGA might have been "immersed in the literature on psychogenic amnesia" ([5], p.4; but see also [221]). The largest reported patient series of TPA in recent times included 53 patients seen over a period of nearly 20 years [217].

TPA may be differentiated from TGA on a number of grounds (Table 3.3) [222]. Attacks tend to be longer, lasting from days to months or even years. The patient's loss of personal identity is a clear differentiating factor of TPA from TGA [217]. Functional amnesias are typically retrograde in nature, with relatively sparing of anterograde memory, hence a reversal of the typical (Ribot) gradient seen in other forms of amnesia, persistent and transient, including TGA [217, 223]. Patients may be far from their home, with no clear history of how they got there (fugue state), sometimes resulting in media coverage to try to identify the individual.

The behavioural disturbances sometimes seen in TGA (Sect. 2.1.2) are generally not a feature of TPA, wherein patients are often not obviously distressed by their amnesia. This may be because they are apparently able to learn new information, despite the dense retrograde amnesia. TPA patients also tend to be younger than patients with TGA.

Once available, there is often a previous history of mood disorder such as depression, and often a clear stressful precipitating event such as relationship or financial problems, and minor head injury. Failure to recognise family members, once located, is common. Spontaneous recovery of memory may occur after a variable time period, with the prognosis for fugue states particularly favourable [217].

The portrayal of characters with amnesia in motion pictures almost invariably features loss of personal identity [224, 225], as seen in TPA, no doubt for dramatic effect.

3.4   Other Symptomatic Causes of Transient Amnesia

Transient amnesia may result from a variety of other conditions and causes (Table 3.2).

3.4.1   Migraine

The possible pathogenic relationship between TGA and migraine is considered in more detail later (Sect. 7.9 and Sect. 9.3). Here, it is simply noted that, amongst the many transient phenomena that may be encountered in the context of migraine attacks, amnesia is sometimes prominent (Case Study 3.3).

Case Study 3.3: Migraine amnesia
A 27-year-old lady was referred to the clinic following a strange experience whilst driving her car. During daylight hours, she set off on the familiar route to her boyfriend's house, part of which involved driving along a motorway. She recollected joining the motorway, but then had no recollection until she found herself six junctions and several miles further on, when she should have turned off after only three junctions. At this point, she stopped to telephone her boyfriend to explain what had happened and that she would be late. On arrival, he noted that she looked shaken, complained of a headache and took some analgesics, but on direct questioning there was no history of repetitive questioning or loss of personal identity. The patient had a prior history of migraine as a teenager, and headaches had recurred some 5 months earlier. Subsequent neurological examination and structural brain imaging were normal. The provisional diagnosis of her "unconscious driving phenomenon" was migraine (adapted from [226]).

Moersch (1924) [227] was perhaps the first to emphasise amnestic dysfunction occurring in migraine attacks. Comorbidity of TGA and migraine was noted in some of the earliest reports of TGA (e.g. [8, 228–230]). Frank (1976) compared amnesic episodes in migraine ("Migranedammerattacken") with reports of TGA and was of the view that they "seem to be identical" [231]. TGA occurring during a migraine attack has been reported by many authors (e.g. [43, 113, 232, 233]. Many of the familial examples of TGA have either migraine comorbidity, or the episodes have occurred at the same time as a migraine (see Sect. 7.9 and Table 7.3). Some authors consider TGA to be simply a form of migraine aura ([234], p.125–30,168). TGA following mild head injury has been suggested to reflect "traumatic migraine" [235].

A syndrome of "acute confusional migraine" is recognised in children [236] which has been noted to have some features akin to TGA (e.g. [237–239]). Both may be examples of what I have ventured to term "cognitive migraine" [240] (see also discussion in [241]).

3.4.2   Adverse Drug Effect

A large number of pharmacological agents, used for both therapeutic and recreational purposes, have on occasion been associated with episodes of transient amnesia with features considered to be akin to those of TGA (Table 3.8).

There are problems with many of these reports. Many predate diagnostic criteria for TGA (e.g. [130, 268]), and/or present atypical clinical features, sometimes denoted as "TGA-like" episodes (e.g. [251, 269]). For example, reports of an association of TGA with marijuana ingestion include an episode of long duration [251] and a case involving a 6-year-old boy [252]. The description of some events labelled as TGA is not particularly convincing [256]. In some instances, it is not clear whether TGA or TEA is being described [257]. For example, a patient treated with intrathecal baclofen for generalised dystonia had events which "met criteria for transient global amnesia, but were unusual because of their frequent recurrence" [243], an observation that prompts concern about the possibility of an epileptic cause. In this context, a case reported by Zeman et al. is of note: following therapeutic infusion of baclofen, the patient developed short periods of global amnesia, accelerated long-term forgetting and persistent autobiographical amnesia, all features seen in TEA [270].

Some of the implicated medications, such as benzodiazepines [229, 246, 250, 268], are known to be associated with anterograde amnesia (e.g. [271, 272]). Indeed, this association was the stimulus, at least in part, which prompted Merriam (1988) to suggest that endogenous benzodiazepines might play a role in the pathogenesis of TGA [222]. Danek et al. explored the role of the benzodiazepine antagonist flumazenil in reversing TGA (n-of-1 trial), with inconclusive outcome [273].

Alcohol may also have been a confounding factor in some reports (e.g. [268]). The reported association with clioquinol use [244, 245] was excluded from the

Table 3.8: Reports of TGA occurring as an adverse drug effect (see text for caveats about some of these reports)

Drug	Reference(s)
Alprostadil (intracavernosal injection)	Maffei et al. (2020) [242]
Baclofen (intrathecal)	Grande et al. (2008) [243]
Clioquinol	Mumenthaler et al. (1979) [244]
	Kaeser (1984) [245]
Diazepam	Gilbert and Benson (1972) [229]
	Mazzucchi et al. (1980) [246]
Digitalis	Greenlee et al. (1975) [130]
Dimethylsulphoxide (DMSO)	Otrock et al. (2008) [247]
Ergots	Pradalier et al. (2000) [43]
	Gil-Martinez and Galiano (2004) [248]
Heparin	Teh et al. (2010) [249]
Lorazepam	Mazzucchi et al. (1980) [246]
	Sandyk (1985) [250]
Marijuana	Stracciari et al. (1999) [251]
	Shukla and Moore (2004) [252]
	Mansour et al. (2014) [253]
Midazolam	Otrock et al. (2008) [247]
Propafenone	Jones et al. (1995) [254]
Rofecoxib	Hirschfeld et al. (2007) [255]
Rosuvastatin	Healy et al. (2009) [256]
Sibutramine	Fu et al. (2010) [257]
Sildenafil (Viagra)	Savitz and Caplan (2002) [258]
	Gandolfo et al. (2003) [259]
	Shihman et al. (2006) [260]
	Marques-Vilallonga et al. (2014) [261]
	Finsterer (2019) [262]
	Lin et al. (2020) [263]
Sumatriptan (Imigran)	Pradalier et al. (2000) [43]
	Lee et al. (2021) [264]
Tadalafil	Schiefer and Sparing (2005) [265]
	Bardes et al. (2008) [266]
	Machado et al. (2010) [267]
Triazolam	Morris and Estes (1987) [268]
Zolpidem	Tsai et al. (2009) [269]

review by Caplan [274] as more likely to reflect a toxic encephalopathy (see Sect. 3.5.1), a conclusion also reached by Hodges ([5], p.10), but other authors seem to have accepted the association as causal ([275], p.84).

The use of opioid and non-opioid analgesia (hydromorphone, ketorolac) may have been a confounding factor in one report of pain-related TGA, although no signs of opioid intoxication were present [276].

The most frequent reports of drug-associated TGA relate to the use of phospho-diesterase type 5 (PDE-5) inhibitors, sildenafil (Viagra) [258–263] and tadalafil [265–267], used for the treatment of erectile dysfunction. Obviously, there is a possible confounding factor here, namely sexual activity which is a reported pre-cipitating factor for TGA (see Sect. 8.4). TGA has also been reported in association with the use of alprostadil (caverject) [242], a prostaglandin analogue administered by intracavernosal injection for erectile dysfunction. The British National Formulary (BNF) does not mention TGA as a side effect for PDE-5 inhibitors, although "mem-ory loss" is listed amongst the "rare or very rare" side effects of tadalafil when used for pulmonary arterial hypertension or erectile dysfunction (bnf.nice.org.uk/drug/tadalafil.html#cautions; accessed 29/07/21).

Medications prescribed for migraine and associated with TGA might be inciden-tal to migraine-related TGA attacks (Sect. 7.9). Such reports are extremely rare despite the high population prevalence of migraine. Pradalier et al. reported a case of TGA associated with the use of subcutaneous injection of sumatriptan and nasal dihydroergotamine [43]. Gil-Martinez and Galiano reported two cases associated with the use of ergotamine and dihydroergotamine, respectively [248]. Lee et al. reported TGA and myocardial infarction (NSTEMI) in a patient given oral sumat-riptan [264], but pain might also be a confounder here (Sect. 8.5). Werner and Woehrle reported triptan overuse as comorbidity in one case in their series of TGA patients [11].

In summary, at best these are anecdotal accounts of a temporal association between drug use and TGA. Few reports include the typical magnetic resonance imaging changes seen in TGA (e.g. [255, 263]). There are, perhaps unsurprisingly, no rechallenge data attempting to corroborate a causal hypothesis. These accounts may therefore simply represent the chance concurrence of unrelated factors.

3.4.3   Hypoglycaemia

Profound hypoglycaemia is a recognised cause of acute amnesia [1]. It has on occa-sion been considered as a possible cause of TGA [228].

Relatively, few cases of amnesia related to hypoglycaemia in the context of dia-betes mellitus and with longitudinal neuropsychological data have been reported (e.g. [277]). Some have evidence of hippocampal lesions on MR brain imaging [278], but these are confluent high signal changes on T2-weighted imaging which are unlike the punctate changes on MR-DWI seen in TGA. A patient seen by the author showed a focal deficit selective for anterograde memory and learning after acute severe hypoglycaemia, which gradually, though incompletely, reversed over a few months, prompting speculation about hippocampal vulnerability to the effects of neuroglycopaenia ([3], p.248 and [279]). Followed up more than 10 years later, the patient had developed an amnesic dementia, with evidence suggesting particular decline over a period of eight months during which he suffered multiple episodes of hypoglycaemia, followed by relative stability of cognition with improvement in gly-caemic control. MR brain imaging showed global atrophy including the medial tem-poral lobes but little in the way of small vessel ischaemic change [280]. There were similarities with the patient reported by Kirchhoff et al. [281] who had multiple hypoglycaemic episodes over many years and whose neuropsychological assessment showed anterograde amnesia; volumetric MR brain imaging showed atrophic change including loss of subcortical grey matter volume involving the hippocampus.

3.4.4 Traumatic Brain (Closed Head) Injury

Patients suffering a traumatic brain injury may present with confusion and memory loss after the injury. The duration of post-traumatic amnesia (PTA) is a marker of head injury severity and is also related to prognosis.

TGA is differentiated from the transient PTA which may follow mild traumatic brain injury (mTBI) secondary to closed head injury by the absence of head injury and the preservation of consciousness. The Hodges and Warlow TGA diagnostic criteria [22] (Table 2.1) list "recent head injury" as an exclusion criterion although "recent" is undefined. Hence, with the availability of a reliable eye-witness account from a capable observer who was present for most of the attack (an inclusion criterion for TGA [22]), there is usually no diagnostic or differential diagnostic issue.

However, in the absence of reliable collateral history, there may be difficulty differentiating PTA and TGA if there are no obvious stigmata of injury, since there is clinical overlap between these transient forms of amnesia. For example, a case of amnesia following mild head injury reported as early as 1835 by Koempfen [282], and cited by Ribot in his classic text on *Disorders of Memory* [283], may have given rise to the mistaken belief that the latter described TGA in the nineteenth century [284]. Miller Fisher's 1966 account of "concussion amnesia" also illustrates a dissociation between amnesia and impaired consciousness, with transient mnestic features akin to TGA (dense anterograde amnesia, retrograde amnesia, recovery within hours with a persistent memory gap) [285]. Although deficits of anterograde memory are documented in PTA, the repetitive questioning and behavioural changes in TGA are not seen, and there may be additional deficits in attentional and executive functions [286, 287]. Transient psychological amnesia (Sect. 3.3) must also enter the differential diagnosis of transient amnesia following a mild head injury [217].

Although cases of TGA triggered by mild head injury (e.g. [230, 235, 288–290]) and "post-traumatic" transient global amnesia have been reported [291], this may have been incidental, since mild head injury is not uncommon. All these reports predate Hodges and Warlow's criteria [22]. Some have atypical features, such as childhood onset (between age 6.5 and 14.5 years [290], or late teenage onset [288]). Nevertheless, Evans stated that "Rare sequelae of seemingly mild head injury include ... TGA" ([292], p.594) and "Mild head injury can rarely trigger TGA, which in children may actually be confusional migraine" ([292], p.597; see Sect. 3.4.1). However, in the context of head injury, the Hodges and Warlow criteria render the term "post-traumatic TGA" [291] an oxymoron.

One apparent exception is the case reported by Venneri et al. [293] in which the clinical and neuropsychological profile was said to be indistinguishable from TGA, albeit the patient's age (27 years) was atypical. Furthermore, the characteristic, although not specific, abnormality seen on diffusion-weighted magnetic resonance imaging in TGA, namely hyperintense lesion(s) in the hippocampal CA1 region, has also been observed in PTA [294].

3.4.5 Alcohol-Induced Amnesia; Korsakoff Syndrome

Acute alcohol intoxication may be associated with amnesia for events occurring during the period of inebriation, indeed currently this may possibly be the most common cause of transient amnesia, perhaps especially in young people. Islands of preserved memory may be reported, hence the description of this amnesia as of "fragmentary" type. Typically, there is no description of anterograde amnesia or repetitive questioning, so the differential diagnosis from TGA is seldom challenging. Confounding factors (recreational drug use, hypoglycaemia, head injury) may also contribute. Longer, "en bloc", alcoholic blackouts lasting days have also been described.

Korsakoff syndrome, associated with thiamine deficiency, which is often but not invariably a consequence of alcohol misuse [295, 296], may be associated with a chronic cognitive syndrome in which dense and persistent anterograde amnesia is prominent (first well described before Korsakoff, e.g. by Robert Lawson in 1878; see [297]). TGA has on occasion been labelled as an acute but transient Korsakoff's syndrome (e.g. [14, 87] and [298], p.38), but this is a misnomer.

3.4.6 Fatigue Amnesia

Cases of amnesia associated with extreme tiredness have been reported [299].

3.5 Other Causes of Acute Cerebral Disorder

Other acute cerebral disorders may sometimes be mistaken for TGA, even when amnesia is not a symptom. TIA is the most prominent example, but other disorders also enter the differential diagnosis (Table 3.2).

3.5.1   Acute Confusional State/Delirium/ Toxic-Metabolic Encephalopathy

Acute confusional state, or delirium, enters the differential diagnosis of TGA since, by definition, one of the phenotypic features of delirium is change in cognition which may include memory deficit (also disorientation, language impairment, perceptual disturbance) not better accounted for by dementia [300]. Impairment of consciousness, a *sine qua non* for the diagnosis of delirium, may be subtle. As infection, metabolic derangements, and adverse drug effects are the most commonly identified precipitating factors for an acute confusional state, the diagnostic label of toxic-metabolic encephalopathy is sometimes used. Some of the reported examples of TGA associated with medication use (Sect. 3.4.2 and Table 3.7) may in fact be examples of toxic-metabolic encephalopathy.

3.5.2   Acute Brain Infections, Including COVID-19

Benon, who described what may have been the earliest reported unequivocal case of TGA in 1909 [301] (see Sect. 1.2), also described amnesia in cases of syphilitic general paresis [302]. Only occasional cases of TGA associated with neurosyphilis have subsequently been reported [303], some ("TGA-like") with MR imaging changes in the limbic system [304].

Other brain infections which have on occasion been reported in association with TGA include encephalitis due to herpes simplex virus [305, 306] or Epstein–Barr virus [307], although the latter case was associated with partial and generalised epileptic seizures so would not fulfil TGA diagnostic criteria. Herpes simplex encephalitis (HSE) usually manifests with fever, headache, behavioural change and impairments of consciousness so should not be confused with TGA, although very occasionally presentation with isolated memory deficit has been reported [308]. Although cognitive recovery occurs in many patients with HSE, sometimes a dense amnesic syndrome may persist. Other, structural, lesions may sometimes masquerade as HSE [309].

Cases of TGA associated with the pandemic of COVID-19 (SARS-CoV-2) have been reported, associated with the infection per se [310], with infection-related acute stroke (suggested to be thrombotic events) [32], and triggered (possibly) by fear of contracting the infection [311]. Werner et al. reported an increased incidence of TGA seen in their hospital in Germany over a 3.5-month period at the beginning of 2020 which they suggested may be a consequence of the emotional stress occasioned by factors such as social distancing, uncertainty about the future and fear of becoming infected with COVID-19 [312].

3.6 Misdiagnosis

As may be evident from the foregoing sections, TGA has a potentially broad differential diagnosis. Hence, although clinical diagnosis is often straightforward in archetypal cases, misdiagnosis of TGA is not unexpected. In a study of 166 episodes of suspected TGA, Werner and Woehrle found an alternative diagnosis or severe comorbidity impacting the occurrence of the amnestic episode in 10.8%. The most important differential diagnosis was stroke [11]. In the author's cohort, in 23/73 (32%) patients referred to the clinic with suspected TGA, the diagnosis could not be sustained, either because of insufficient clinical evidence (most often the absence of a reliable witness report of the episode) or because an alternative diagnosis was established (see Figure 7.3).

3.7 Summary and Recommendations

The relatively stereotyped clinical features of TGA may render diagnosis straightforward, especially for those clinicians who are familiar with the condition. Nevertheless, acute amnesic episodes have a potentially extensive differential diagnosis, including disorders of cerebrovascular, epileptic, psychological, metabolic, infective, toxic and structural origin. For this reason, investigations may sometimes be required to assist with the diagnosis and differential diagnosis of TGA, and these are elaborated on the next two chapters.

References

1. Fisher CM. Unexplained sudden amnesia. Arch Neurol. 2002;59:1310–3.
2. Papanicolaou AC. The amnesias: a clinical textbook of memory disorders. Oxford: Oxford University Press; 2006.
3. Larner AJ. Dementia in clinical practice: a neurological perspective. In: Pragmatic studies in the cognitive function clinic. 3rd ed. London: Springer; 2018.
4. Larner AJ. Transient global amnesia in the district general hospital. Int J Clin Pract. 2007;61:255–8.
5. Hodges JR. Transient amnesia. Clinical and neuropsychological aspects. London: WB Saunders; 1991.
6. Williamson J, Larner AJ. Transient global amnesia. Br J Hosp Med. 2015;76:C186-8.
7. Guyotat MM, Courjon J. Les ictus amnésiques. J Med Lyon. 1956;37:697–701.
8. Poser CM, Ziegler DK. Temporary amnesia as a manifestation of cerebrovascular insufficiency. Trans Am Neurol Assoc. 1960;85:221–3.
9. Halsey JH Jr. Cerebral infarction with transient global amnesia. Ala J Med Sci. 1967;4:436–8.
10. Fisher CM, Adams RD. Transient global amnesia. Acta Neurol Scand. 1964;40(Suppl9):1–81.
11. Werner R, Woehrle JC. Prevalence of mimics and severe comorbidity in patients with clinically suspected transient global amnesia. Cerebrovasc Dis. 2021;50:171–7.

12. Papez JW. A proposed mechanism of emotion. Arch Neurol Psychiatry. 1937;38:725–43. [Reprinted in J Neuropsychiatry Clin Neurosci. 1995;7:103-12.]
13. Lou H. Repeated episodes of transient global amnesia. Acta Neurol Scand. 1968;44:612–8.
14. de Tribolet N, Assal G, Oberson R. Korsakoff's syndrome and transitory cortical blindness following vertebral angiography [in German]. Schweiz Med Wochenschr. 1975;105:1506–9.
15. Benson DF, Marsden CD, Meadows JC. The amnesic syndrome of posterior cerebral artery occlusion. Acta Neurol Scand. 1974;50:133–45.
16. Howard RS, Festenstein R, Mellers J, Kartsounis LD, Ron M. Transient amnesia heralding brain stem infarction. J Neurol Neurosurg Psychiatry. 1992;55:977.
17. Taylor RA, Wu GF, Hurst RW, Kasner SE, Cucchiara BL. Transient global amnesia heralding basilar artery thrombosis. Clin Neurol Neurosurg. 2005;108:60–2.
18. Carota A, Lysandropoulos AP, Calabrese P. Pure left hippocampal stroke: a transient global amnesia-plus syndrome. J Neurol. 2012;259:989–92.
19. Beyrouti R, Mansour M, Kacem A, Zaouali J, Mrissa R. Transient global amnesia like syndrome associated with acute infarction of the corpus callosum: a case report. Acta Neurol Belg. 2016;116:375–7.
20. Michel P, Beaud V, Eskandari A, Maeder P, Demonet JF, Eskioglou E. Ischemic amnesia: causes and outcome. Stroke. 2017;48:2270–3.
21. Ott BR, Saver JL. Unilateral amnesic stroke. Six new cases and a review of the literature. Stroke. 1993;24:1033–42.
22. Hodges JR, Warlow CP. Syndromes of transient amnesia: towards a classification. A study of 153 cases. J Neurol Neurosurg Psychiatry. 1990;53:834–43.
23. Chen ST, Tang LM, Lee TH, Ro LS, Lyu RK. Transient global amnesia and amaurosis fugax in a patient with common carotid artery occlusion—a case report. Angiology. 2000;51:257–61.
24. Bogousslavsky J, Regli F. Transient global amnesia and stroke. Eur Neurol. 1988;28:106–10.
25. Gorelick PB, Amico LL, Ganellen R, Benevento LA. Transient global amnesia and thalamic infarction. Neurology. 1988;38:496–9.
26. Raffaele R, Tornali C, Genazzani AA, Vecchio I, Rampello L. Transient global amnesia and cerebral infarct: a case report. Brain Inj. 1995;9:815–8.
27. Larner AJ. Stroke as a cause of TGA? Narrative review and hypothesis. J Neurol Disord Stroke. 2022;9(1):1189.
28. Greer DM, Schaefer PW, Schwamm LH. Unilateral temporal lobe stroke causing ischemic transient global amnesia: role for diffusion-weighted imaging in the initial evaluation. J Neuroimaging. 2001;11:317–9.
29. López-Pesquera B, Fratalia-Bax L, Piera-Balbastre A, Badia-Picazo MC, Chamarro LR. Amnesia global transitoria. No siempre un proceso benigno. Rev Neurol. 2005;41:57. (Poster P7)
30. Graff-Radford J, Clapp AJ, Lanzino G, Rabinstein AA. Transient amnesia after coiling of a posterior circulation aneurysm. Neurocrit Care. 2013;18:245–7.
31. Duan H, Li L, Zhang Y, Zhang J, Chen M, Bao S. Transient global amnesia following neural and cardiac angiography may be related to ischemia. Biomed Res Int. 2016;2016:2821765.
32. Ramanathan RS, Wachsman A. Coronavirus disease-19 (COVID-19) related acute stroke causing transient global amnesia. J Stroke Cerebrovasc Dis. 2021;30:105738.
33. Adler AC, Warum D, Sapire JM. Transient global amnesia caused by hippocampal infarct: case report and review of literature. Clin Imaging. 2012;36:584–6.
34. Gungor-Tuncer O, Okudan Z, Aksay-Koyuncu B, Altindag E, Tolun R, Krespi Y. Posterior circulation stroke: an underdiagnosed situation in transient global amnesia. J Neurol. 2012;259(Suppl1):S115. (abstract P484)
35. Gungor Tuncer O, Aksay Koyuncu B, Vildan Okudan Z, Altindag E, Tolun R, Krespi Y. Vascular ischemia as a cause of transient global amnesia: a patient series. Noro Psikiyatr Ars. 2015;52:59–63.
36. Li J, Hu WL. Bilateral hippocampal abnormalities in magnetic resonance imaging in transient global amnesia. Am J Emerg Med. 2013;31:755e1–3.

37. Naldi F, Baiardi S, Guarino M, Spinardi L, Cirignotta F, Stracciari A. Posterior hippocampal stroke presenting with transient global amnesia. Neurocase. 2016;23:22–5.
38. Yun U, Hwang I, Ha SW. Transient global amnesia caused by bilateral medial temporal-lobe infarction. Dement Neurocogn Disord. 2017;16:132–3.
39. Kang MK, Kim SY, Kang HG, Shin BS, Lee CH. Transient global amnesia caused by cryptogenic ischemic stroke. Interdiscip Neurosurg. 2021;23:100911.
40. Sakihara E, Ajisaka K, Takeoka H, Suzuyama H, Nabeshima S. A case of transient global amnesia with hippocampal infarction due to infective endocarditis. J Infect Chemother. 2021;27:902–5.
41. Gupta M, Kantor MA, Tung CE, Zhang N, Albers GW. Transient global amnesia associated with a unilateral infarction of the fornix: case report and review of the literature. Front Neurol. 2015;5:291.
42. Meyer MA. Neurologic disease. A modern pathophysiologic approach to diagnosis and treatment. London: Springer; 2016.
43. Pradalier A, Lutz G, Vincent D. Transient global amnesia, migraine, thalamic infarct, dihydroergotamine, and sumatriptan. Headache. 2000;40:324–7.
44. Giannantoni NM, Lacidogna G, Broccolini A, et al. Thalamic amnesia mimicking transient global amnesia. Neurologist. 2015;19:149–52.
45. Dogan VB, Dogan GB, Turkmen U, Yayla VA. A case of thalamo-mesencephalon infarct presenting as transient global amnesia: do we overlook the diagnosis? Neurol Sci. 2017;38:909–11.
46. Gallardo-Tur A, Romero-Godoy J, de la Cruz Cosme C, Arboix A. Transient global amnesia associated with an acute infarction at the cingulate gyrus. Case Rep Neurol Med. 2014;2014:418180.
47. Chau L, Liu A. Transient global amnesia as the sole presentation of an acute stroke in the left cingulate gyrus. Case Rep Neurol Med. 2019;2019:4810629.
48. Meng D, Alsaeed M, Randhawa J, Chen T. Retrosplenial stroke mimicking transient global amnesia. Can J Neurol Sci. 2021;48:884–5.
49. Ravindran V, Jain S, Ming A, Bartlett RJ. Transient global amnesia in a patient with acute unilateral caudate nucleus ischemia. J Clin Neurosci. 2004;11:669–72.
50. Kim HJ, Kim H, Lim SM, Moon WJ, Han SH. An acute tiny left putamenal lesion presenting with transient global amnesia. Neurologist. 2012;18:80–2.
51. Koltermann T, Vitali da Silva A, Pires Lazaro Fay Neves M, Parizotto C, da Silva J, Batista de Rezende Filho O. Case report: caudate stroke simulating transient global amnesia. J Neurol Sci. 2015;357(Suppl1):e387–8.
52. Yoshida K. A case of transient global amnesia with small left putamen infarction. J Stroke Cerebrovasc Dis. 2017;26:e27-8.
53. Tarazona LR, Martinez EL, Llopis CM. Transient global amnesia with extra-hippocampal lesion and a normal cardiovascular study. Can J Neurol Sci. 2021;24:1–2. https://doi.org/10.1017/cjn.2021.116. Online ahead of print.
54. Saito K, Kimura K, Minematsu K, Shiraishi A, Nakajima M. Transient global amnesia associated with an acute infarction in the retrosplenium of the corpus callosum. J Neurol Sci. 2003;210:95–7.
55. Kim J, Sohn MJ, Choi SW. Acute ischemic strokes presenting as transient global amnesia. Eur J Neurol. 2018;25(Suppl2):106. (abstract EPO1032)
56. Chatham PE, Brillman J. Transient global amnesia associated with bilateral subdural hematomas. Neurosurgery. 1985;17:971–3.
57. Heon M, Reiher D, Dilenge D, Lamarche J. Ictus amnésique et hématome intraventriculaire. Neuro-chirurgie (Paris). 1972;18:503–10.
58. Honma Y, Nagao S. Hemorrhagic pituitary adenoma manifesting as transient global amnesia. Neurol Med Chir (Tokyo). 1996;36:234–6.
59. Jacome DE, Yanez GF. Transient global amnesia and left frontal haemorrhage. Postgrad Med J. 1988;64:137–9.

60. Landi G, Giusti MC, Guidotti M. Transient global amnesia due to left temporal haemorrhage. J Neurol Neurosurg Psychiatry. 1982;45:1062–3.
61. Monzani V, Rovellini A, Schinco G, Silani V. Transient global amnesia or subarachnoid haemorrhage? Clinical and laboratory findings in a particular type of acute global amnesia. Eur J Emerg Med. 2000;7:291–3.
62. Moonis M, Jain S, Prasad K, Mishra NK, Goulatia RK, Maheshwari MC. Left thalamic hypertensive haemorrhage presenting as transient global amnesia. Acta Neurol Scand. 1988;77:331–4.
63. Sandyk R. Transient global amnesia: a presentation of subarachnoid haemorrhage. J Neurol. 1984;231:283–4.
64. Sorenson EJ, Silbert PL, Benarroch EE, Jack CR, Parisi JE. Transient amnesic syndrome after spontaneous haemorrhage into a hypothalamic pilocytic astrocytoma. J Neurol Neurosurg Psychiatry. 1995;58:761–3.
65. Yoon B, Yoo JY, Shim YS, Lee KS, Kim JS. Transient global amnesia associated with acute intracerebral haemorrhage at the cingulate gyrus. Eur Neurol. 2006;56:54–6.
66. Wilson M, Doran M, Enevoldson TP, Larner AJ. Cognitive profiles associated with intracranial dural arteriovenous fistula. Age Ageing. 2010;39:389–92.
67. Randall A, Ellis R, Hywel B, Davies RR, Alusi SH, Larner AJ. Rapid cognitive decline: not always Creutzfeldt-Jakob disease. J R Coll Physicians Edinb. 2015;45:209–12.
68. Johnson P, Ghodke B, Khot S. Dural arteriovenous fistula causing recurrent transient global amnesia. Neurohospitalist. 2018;8:200.
69. Takahashi Y, Yamamoto T, Abe T, et al. Transient global amnesia and dural arteriovenous fistula of the anterior cranial fossa. Kurume Med J. 1996;43:223–9.
70. Heine P, Degos JD, Meyrignac C. Cerebral angioma disclosed by 2 episodes of transient global amnesia [in French]. Presse Med. 1986;15:1049.
71. Daniel BT. Transient global amnesia. Print version and ebook: Amazon; 2012.
72. Boitet R, Gaillard N, Bendiab E, et al. Concomitant reversible cerebral vasoconstriction syndrome and transient global amnesia. J Neurol. 2020;267:390–4.
73. Ishaya K, Shinohara K, Akamatu M, et al. Reversible cerebral vasoconstriction syndrome presenting with transient global amnesia. Intern Med. 2017;56:1569–73.
74. Kamm K, Schöberl F, Grabova D, Straube A, Zwergal A. RCVS and TGA: a common pathophysiology? J Neurol. 2019;266:2872–4.
75. Kim J, Jung YI, Seo J, Lee H, Sunwoo MK. A case of posterior reversible encephalopathy syndrome with similar symptoms as transient global amnesia. Dement Neurocogn Disord. 2018;17:176–8.
76. Nakamizo T, Tsuzuki I, Koide T. Transient global amnesia with reversible white matter lesions: a variant of posterior reversible encephalopathy syndrome? Case Rep Neurol Med. 2015;2015:541328.
77. Rumpl E, Rumpl H. Recurrent transient global amnesia in a case with cerebrovascular lesions and livedo reticularis (Sneddon syndrome). J Neurol. 1979;221:127–31.
78. Nishida A, Kaiya H, Uematsu M, Maeda M, Mori S, Wakabayashi S. Transient global amnesia and Raynaud's phenomenon in scleroderma. Acta Neurol Scand. 1990;81:550–2.
79. Pradotto L, Orsi L, Mencarelli M, et al. Recurrent transient global amnesia as presenting symptoms of CADASIL. Clin Case Rep. 2016;4:1045–8.
80. Garcia-Carrasco M, Galarza C, Gomez-Ponce M, et al. Antiphospholipid syndrome in Latin American patients: clinical and immunologic characteristics and comparison with European patients. Lupus. 2007;16:366–73.
81. Ortego-Centeno N, Callejas-Rubio JL, Fernandez MG, Carmello MG. Transient global amnesia in a patient with high and persistent levels of antiphospholipid antibodies. Clin Rheumatol. 2006;25:407–8.
82. Cervera R, Piette JC, Font J, et al. Antiphospholipid syndrome: clinical and immunologic manifestations and patterns of disease expression in a cohort of 1,000 patients. Arthritis Rheum. 2002;46:1019–27.

83. Attarian S, Michel B, Delaforte C, Chave B, Gastaut JL. A case of transient amnesia caused by cerebral thrombophlebitis: contribution of neuroimaging to physiopathogenesis of transient amnesia [in French]. Rev Neurol (Paris). 1995;151:552–8.

84. Sharma RC, Kainth A, Sharma S. Transient global amnesia as a presenting manifestation of cerebral venous thrombosis. J Neuropsychiatry Clin Neurosci. 2015;27:e209–10.

85. Ito AO, Tamura A, Niwa A, et al. Recurrent transient global amnesia associated with internal jugular vein thrombosis. J Neurol Sci. 2019;402:108–10.

86. Hauge T. Catheter vertebral angiography. Acta Radiologica Suppl. 1954;109:1–219.

87. Deak G, Toth S. Vertebral angiography followed by transient Korsakoff's syndrome [in Hungarian]. Ideggyogy Sz. 1964;17:119–25.

88. Whishart DL. Complications of cerebral angiography as compared to non-vertebral cerebral angiography in 447 studies. AJR Am J Roentgenol. 1971;113:527–37.

89. Wales LR, Nov AA. Transient global amnesia: complication of cerebral angiography. AJN R Am J Neuroradiol. 1981;2:275–7.

90. Cochran JW, Morrell F, Huckman MS, Cochran EJ. Transient global amnesia after cerebral angiography. Report of seven cases. Arch Neurol. 1982;39:593–4.

91. Haas DC. Transient global amnesia after cerebral angiography. Arch Neurol. 1983;40:258–9.

92. Pexman JH, Coates RK. Amnesia after femorocerebral angiography. AJNR Am J Neuroradiol. 1983;4:979–83.

93. Giang DW, Kido DK. Transient global amnesia associated with cerebral angiography performed with use of iopamidol. Radiology. 1989;172:195–6.

94. Minuk J, Melancon D, Tampieri D, Ethier R. Transient global amnesia associated with cerebral angiography performed with use of iopamidol. Radiology. 1990;174:285–6.

95. Juni J, Morera J, Lainez JM, Escudero J, Ferrer C, Sancho J. Transient global amnesia after cerebral angiography with iohexol. Neuroradiology. 1992;34:141–3.

96. Brady AP, Hough DM, Lo R, Gill G. Transient global amnesia after cerebral angiography with iohexol. Can Assoc Radiol J. 1993;44:450–2.

97. Schamschula RG, Soo MY. Transient global amnesia following cerebral angiography with non-ionic contrast medium. Australas Radiol. 1994;38:196–8.

98. Jackson A, Stewart G, Wood A, Gillespie JE. Transient global amnesia and cortical blindness after vertebral angiography: further evidence for the role of arterial spasm. AJNR Am J Neuroradiol. 1995;16(4Suppl):955–9.

99. Meder JF, Mourey-Gerosa I, Blustain J, Lemaignen H, Devaux B, Fredy D. Transient global amnesia after cerebral angiography. A case report. Acta Radiol. 1997;38:273–4.

100. Woolfenden AR, O'Brien MW, Schwartzberg RE, Norbash AM, Tong DC. Diffusion-weighted MRI in transient global amnesia precipitated by cerebral angiography. Stroke. 1997;28:2311–4.

101. Kapur N, Millar J, Abbott P, Carter M. Recovery of function processes in human amnesia: evidence from transient global amnesia. Neuropsychologia. 1998;36:99–107.

102. Tanabe M, Watanabe T, Ishibashi M, Hirano M, Tabuchi S, Takigawa H. Hippocampal ischemia in a patient who experienced transient global amnesia after undergoing cerebral angiography. Case illustration. J Neurosurg. 1999;91:347.

103. Kim HY, Kang HS, Roh HG, Oh J, Lee IK, Han SH. Transient global amnesia following vertebral artery angioplasty and stenting. Eur Neurol. 2006;56:133–5.

104. Foss-Skiftesvik J, Snoer AH, Wagner A, Hauerberg J. Transient global amnesia after cerebral angiography still occurs: case report and literature review. Radiol Case Rep. 2015;9:988.

105. Tiu C, Terecoasa EO, Grecu N, Dorobat B, Marinescu AN, Bajenaru OA. Transient global amnesia after cerebral angiography with iomeprol: a case report. Medicine (Baltimore). 2016;95:e3950.

106. Lee BH. Transient global amnesia following carotid artery stenting: a case report. Radiol Case Rep. 2020;15:1159–63.

107. Fischer-Williams M, Gottschalk PG, Browell JN. Transient cortical blindness. An unusual complication of coronary angiography. Neurology. 1970;29:353–5.

108. Shuttleworth EC, Wise GR. Transient global amnesia due to arterial embolism. Arch Neurol. 1973;29:340–2.
109. Lockwood K, Capraro J, Hanson M, Conomy J. Neurologic complications of cardiac catheterization. Neurology. 1983;33(Suppl2):143.
110. Koehler PJ, Endtz LJ, den Bakker PB. Transient global amnesia after coronary angiography. Clin Cardiol. 1986;9:170–1.
111. Yildiz A, Yencilek E, Apaydin FD, Duce MN, Ozer C, Atalay A. Transient partial amnesia complicating cardiac and peripheral arteriography with nonionic contrast medium. Eur Radiol. 2003;13(Suppl4):L113-5.
112. Kurokawa Y, Ishizaki E, Kihara H, Inaba K. Two cases of transient global amnesia (TGA) immediately after coronary angiography: pathogenesis of the primary TGA [in Japanese]. No To Shinkei. 2004;56:69–74.
113. Fernandez A, Rincon F, Mazer SP, Elkind MS. Magnetic resonance imaging changes in a patient with migraine attack and transient global amnesia after cardiac catheterization. CNS Spectr. 2005;10:980–3.
114. Wong E, Patel A, Javasinghe R. Transient global amnesia following coronary angiography and angioplasty. Intern Med J. 2005;37:435–6.
115. Udyavar AR, D'souza RC, Gadkar N, Rajani RM. Transient global amnesia following coronary angiography. J Postgrad Med. 2006;52:70–1.
116. Rosenberg GA. Transient global amnesia with a dissecting aortic aneurysm. Arch Neurol. 1979;36:255.
117. Gaul C, Dietrich W, Tomandi B, Neundörfer B, Erbguth FJ. Aortic dissection presenting with transient global amnesia-like symptoms. Neurology. 2004;63:2442–3.
118. Mondon K, Blechet C, Gochard A, et al. Transient global amnesia caused by painless aortic dissection. Emerg Med J. 2007;24:63–4.
119. Irioka T, Yamanami A, Yaqi Y, Mizusawa H. Aortic dissection as a possible cause of pure transient global amnesia: a case report and literature review. Neurol Sci. 2009;30:255–8.
120. Colotto M, Maranghi M, Epifania A, Totaro M, Giura R, Durante C. Unmasking aortic dissection in patients of [sic] transient global amnesia: case report and diagnostic algorithm for the emergency department. BMJ Case Rep. 2011;2011:pii:bcr0720103151.
121. Kaveeshvar H, Kashouty R, Loomba V, Yono N. A rare case of aortic dissection presenting as pure transient global amnesia. Cardiovasc J Afr. 2015;26:e8–9.
122. Michel D, Garnier P, Schneider F, Poujois A, Barral FG, Thomas-Antérion C. Diffusion MRI in pure transient global amnesia associated with bilateral vertebral artery dissection. Cerebrovasc Dis. 2004;17:264–6.
123. Yokota H, Yokoyama K, Iwasaki S. Transient global amnesia with intracranial vertebral artery dissection and hippocampal CA1 lesion. Neurol India. 2015;63:604–5.
124. Renault P, Rouchet S. Transient global amnesia and transient cortical blindness secondary to contrast induced encephalopathy after renal artery angiography. Rev Neurol (Paris). 2019;175:335–6.
125. Hankey GJ. Recurrent migraine aura triggered by coronary angiography. Pract Neurol. 2004;4:308–9.
126. Agosti C, Borroni B, Akkawi N, Bordonali T, Padovani A. Acute myocardial infarction presenting with transient global amnesia spectrum. J Am Geriatr Soc. 2006;54:1004.
127. Caramelli B, Dutra AP, Calderaro D, Yu PC, Gualandro DM, Marques AC. Transient global amnesia as a manifestation of acute myocardial infarction: a case of missed sudden cardiac death? Int J Cardiol. 2009;136:e14–5.
128. Courand PY, Sibellas F, Gonidec S, Mechtouff L, Kirkorian G, Bonnefoy E. Acute myocardial infarction: a precipitating event for transient global amnesia. J Cardiovasc Med (Hagerstown). 2014;15:78–9.
129. Harase S, Araki K, Kobayashi T, Katada F, Fukutake T. A case of transient global amnesia associated with painless myocardial infarction [in Japanese]. Rinsho Shinkeigaku. 2021;61:136–9.

130. Greenlee JE, Crampton RS, Miller JQ. Transient global amnesia associated with cardiac arrhythmia and digitalis intoxication. Stroke. 1975;6:513–6.
131. Ullrich NJ, Urion DK. Transient global amnesia in a young adult with cyanotic heart disease. Pediatr Neurol. 2003;29:334–6.
132. Jackson AC. Neurologic disorders associated with mitral valve prolapse. Can J Neurol Sci. 1986;13:15–20.
133. Bobinger T, Köhrmann M, Raaz-Schrauder D, Schwab S, Kallmünzer B. Lost memories can break your heart: a case report of transient global amnesia followed by takotsubo cardiomyopathy. Clin Res Cardiol. 2013;102:693–6.
134. Eisele P, Baumann S, Noor L, et al. Interaction between the heart and the brain in transient global amnesia. J Neurol. 2019;266:3048–57.
135. Finsterer J, Stöllberger C. Simultaneous transient global amnesia and Takotsubo syndrome after death of a relative: a case report. J Med Case Rep. 2019;13(1):22.
136. Grautoff S, Sitzer M, Weitkamp P, Kähler J. Transient global amnesia and Tako-Tsubo cardiomyopathy—coincidence or corollary? [in German]. Dtsch Med Wochenschr. 2012;137:2256–9.
137. Petrea RE, Nguyen T, Pikula A, Wilkenfeld A, Nedeljkovic Z, Kase CS. Transient global amnesia heralding a broken-heart syndrome. Eur J Neurol. 2008;15(Suppl3):212–3. (abstract P1718)
138. Pyle LM, Laghari FJ, Kinem DJ. Concomitant transient global amnesia and takotsubo cardiomyopathy following a stressful event. Clin Auton Res. 2018;28:597–8.
139. Quick S, Speiser U, Richter N, et al. Transient global amnesia and broken heart syndrome: two faces of one pathology. Clin Auton Res. 2015;25:189–91.
140. Sajeev J, Koshy A, Rajakariar K, Gordon G. Takotsubo cardiomyopathy and transient global amnesia: a shared aetiology. BMJ Case Rep. 2017;2017:bcr2017219472.
141. Stöllberger C, DeCilla N, Finsterer J. Tako-tsubo cardiomyopathy with transient global amnesia and cerebellar embolic stroke triggered by existential fear. Neurol Neurochir Pol. 2018;52:394–6.
142. Tso M, Tam JW, Khoo C. An atypical case of Takotsubo cardiomyopathy and transient global amnesia. CJC Open. 2019;1:35–8.
143. Pelliccia F, Parodi G, Greco C, et al. Comorbidities frequency in Takotsubo syndrome: an international collaborative systematic review including 1109 patients. Am J Med. 2015;128(654):e11–9.
144. Finsterer J, Stöllberger C. Transient global amnesia: the cerebral Takotsubo? J Neurol Sci. 2017;376:196–7.
145. Erdur H, Siegerink B, Ganeshan R, et al. Myocardial injury in transient global amnesia: a case-control study. Eur J Neurol. 2019;26:986–91.
146. Jaguszewski M, Osipova J, Ghadri JR, et al. A signature of circulating microRNAs differentiates Takotsubo cardiomyopathy from acute myocardial infarction. Eur Heart J. 2014;35:999–1006.
147. Klötzsch C, Sliwka U, Berlit P, Noth J. An increased frequency of patent foramen ovale in patients with transient global amnesia. Analysis of 53 consecutive patients. Arch Neurol. 1996;53:504–8.
148. Profice P, Rizzello V, Pennestri F, et al. Transient global amnesia during transoesophageal echocardiogram. Neurol Sci. 2008;29:477–9.
149. Maalikjy Akkawi N, Agosti C, Anzola GP, et al. Transient global amnesia: a clinical and sonographic study. Eur Neurol. 2003;49:67–71.
150. Noh SM, Kang HG. Clinical manifestation and imaging characteristics of transient global amnesia: patent foramen ovale as an underlying factor. J Integr Neurosci. 2021;20:719–25.
151. Spigno F, De Lucchi M, Migliazzi L, Cocito L. Transient global amnesia after breathing hyperoxic mixtures in otherwise regular dives. Clin Neurol Neurosurg. 2008;110:259–61.
152. Liu K, Wang BZ, Hao Y, Song S, Pan M. The correlation between migraine and patent foramen ovale. Front Neurol. 2020;11:543485.

153. Deisenhammer E. Transient global amnesia as an epileptic manifestation. J Neurol. 1981;225:289–92.
154. Gilbert GJ. Transient global amnesia: manifestation of medial temporal lobe epilepsy. Clin Electroencephalogr. 1978;9:147–52.
155. Melo TP, Ferro JM, Paiva T. Are brief or recurrent transient global amnesias of epileptic origin? J Neurol Neurosurg Psychiatry. 1994;57:622–5.
156. Meo R, Bilo L, Striano S, Ruosi P, Estraneo A, Nocerino C. Transient global amnesia of epileptic origin accompanied by fever. Seizure. 1995;4:311–7.
157. Tharp BR. Transient global amnesia: manifestation of medial temporal lobe epilepsy. Clin Electroencephalogr. 1979;10:54–6.
158. Fisher CM. Transient global amnesia. Precipitating activities and other observations. Arch Neurol. 1982;39:605–8.
159. Caplan LR. C. Miller Fisher. Stroke in the 20th century. New York: Oxford University Press; 2020.
160. Fisher CM. Ataxic hemiparesis. A pathologic study. Arch Neurol. 1978;35:126–8.
161. Fisher CM. Pure sensory stroke and allied conditions. Stroke. 1982;13:434–47.
162. Werring D, Greenberg SM, Gill S. Foundations of modern stroke medicine. The legacy of C Miller Fisher. Adv Clin Neurosci Rehabil. 2015;15(5):18–9.
163. Jackson JH. On a particular variety of epilepsy (intellectual aura). One case with symptoms of organic brain disease. Brain. 1888;11:179–207.
164. Gallassi R, Morreale A, Lorusso S, Pazzaglia P, Lugaresi E. Epileptic transient amnesia. Ital J Neurol Sci. 1988;(Suppl 9):37–9.
165. Gallassi R, Morreale A, Di Sarro R, Lugaresi E. Epileptic amnesic syndrome. Epilepsia. 1992;33(suppl6):S21–5.
166. Palmini AL, Gloor P, Jones-Gotman M. Pure amnestic seizures in temporal lobe epilepsy. Definition, clinical symptomatology and functional anatomical considerations. Brain. 1992;115:749–69.
167. Pritchard PB III, Holmstrom VL, Roitzsch JC, Giacinto J. Epileptic amnesic attacks: benefit from antiepileptic drugs. Neurology. 1985;35:1188–9.
168. Rowan AJ, Rosenbaum DH. Ictal amnesia and fugue states. Adv Neurol. 1991;55:357–67.
169. Stracciari A, Ciucci G, Bianchedi G, Rebucci GG. Epileptic transient amnesia. Eur Neurol. 1990;30:176–9.
170. Kapur N. Transient epileptic amnesia: a clinical update and a reformulation. J Neurol Neurosurg Psychiatry. 1993;56:1184–90.
171. Zeman AZJ, Boniface SJ, Hodges JR. Transient epileptic amnesia: a description of the clinical and neuropsychological features in 10 cases and a review of the literature. J Neurol Neurosurg Psychiatry. 1998;64:435–43.
172. Asadi-Pooya AA. Transient epileptic amnesia: a concise review. Epilepsy Behav. 2014;31:243–5.
173. Baker J, Savage S, Milton F, et al. The syndrome of transient epileptic amnesia: a combined series of 115 cases and literature review. Brain Commun. 2021;3:fcab038.
174. Bartsch T, Butler C. Transient amnesic syndromes. Nat Rev Neurol. 2013;9:86–97.
175. Butler C. Transient epileptic amnesia. Pract Neurol. 2006;6:368–71.
176. Butler CR, Zeman AZ. Recent insights into the impairment of memory in epilepsy: transient epileptic amnesia, accelerated long-term forgetting and remote memory impairment. Brain. 2008;131:2243–63.
177. Butler CR, Zeman A. The causes and consequences of transient epileptic amnesia. Behav Neurol. 2011;24:299–305.
178. Butler CR, Graham KS, Hodges JR, Kapur N, Wardlaw JM, Zeman AZ. The syndrome of transient epileptic amnesia. Ann Neurol. 2007;61:587–98.
179. Ramanan VK, Morris KA, Graff-Radford J, et al. Transient epileptic amnesia: a treatable cause of spells associated with persistent cognitive symptoms. Front Neurol. 2019;10:939.

180. Zeman A, Butler C, Hodges J, Kapur N. The syndrome of transient epileptic amnesia. In: Zeman A, Kapur N, Jones-Gotman M, editors. Epilepsy and memory. Oxford: Oxford University Press; 2012. p. 139–59.

181. Manes F, Hodges JR, Graham KS, et al. Focal autobiographical amnesia in association with transient epileptic amnesia. Brain. 2001;124:499–509.

182. Manes F, Graham KS, Zeman A, de Luján Calcagno M, Hodges JR. Autobiographical amnesia and accelerated forgetting in transient epileptic amnesia. J Neurol Neurosurg Psychiatry. 2005;76:1387–91.

183. Blake R, Wroe S, Breen E, McCarthy R. Accelerated forgetting in patients with epilepsy: evidence for impairment in memory consolidation. Brain. 2000;123:472–83.

184. McGinty RN, Larner AJ. Transient epileptic amnesia and pathological tearfulness. Cortex. 2022;147:206–8.

185. Felician O, Tramoni E, Barbeau E, et al. Isolated autobiographical amnesia: a neurological basis? [in French]. Rev Neurol (Paris). 2009;165:449–59.

186. Kapur N. Focal retrograde amnesia in neurological disease: a critical review. Cortex. 1993;29:217–34.

187. Larner AJ, Ghadiali EJ, Doran M. Focal retrograde amnesia: clinical, neuropsychological and neuroimaging study. Neurobiol Aging. 2004;25(S2):S128. (abstract P1-116)

188. Stuss DT, Guzman DA. Severe remote memory loss with minimal anterograde amnesia: a clinical note. Brain Cogn. 1988;8:21–30.

189. Lozsadi DA, Chadwick DW, Larner AJ. Late-onset temporal lobe epilepsy with unilateral mesial temporal sclerosis and cognitive decline: a diagnostic dilemma. Seizure. 2008;17:473–6.

190. Butler C, van Erp W, Bhaduri A, Hammers A, Heckemann R, Zeman A. Magnetic resonance volumetry reveals focal brain atrophy in transient epileptic amnesia. Epilepsy Behav. 2013;28:363–9.

191. Kanbayahsi T, Hatanaka Y, Sonoo M. Transient epileptic amnesia with amygdala enlargement. Neurol Sci. 2020;41:1591–3.

192. Larner AJ. Transient epileptic amnesia and amygdala enlargement revisited. Psychogeriatrics. 2021;21:943–4.

193. Takeda M, Kasama S, Watanabe S, Kimura T, Yoshikawa H. Transient epileptic amnesia in a temporal lobe epilepsy patient with amygdala enlargement: a case study. Psychogeriatrics. 2020;20:235–6.

194. Milburn-McNulty P, Larner AJ. Transient global amnesia and brain tumour: chance concurrence or aetiological association? Case report and systematic literature review. Case Rep Neurol. 2015;7:18–25.

195. Krishnan K, Larner AJ. Concurrent onset of transient epileptic amnesia and Alzheimer's disease. Eur J Neurol. 2009;16(Suppl 3):468. (abstract 2386)

196. Lozsadi DA, Larner AJ. Prevalence and causes of seizures at time of diagnosis of probable Alzheimer's disease. Dement Geriatr Cogn Disord. 2006;22:121–4.

197. Adan G, Mitchell JW, Ziso B, Larner AJ. Diagnosis and management of seizures in neurodegenerative diseases. Curr Treat Options Neurol. 2021;23:1.

198. Larner AJ. Epileptic seizures in AD patients. Neuromolecular Med. 2010;12:71–7.

199. Larner AJ. Something in common: Alzheimer's disease and epilepsy. EP Epilepsy Prof. 2011;21:12–5.

200. Powell G, Ziso B, Larner AJ. The overlap between epilepsy and Alzheimer's disease and the consequences for treatment. Expert Rev Neurother. 2019;19:653–61.

201. Rabinowicz AL, Starkstein SE, Leiguarda RC, Coleman AE. Transient epileptic amnesia in dementia: a treatable unrecognized cause of episodic amnestic wandering. Alzheimer Dis Assoc Disord. 2000;14:231–3.

202. Huang CF, Pai MC. Transient amnesia in a patient with left temporal tumor. Symptomatic transient global amnesia or an epileptic amnesia? Neurologist. 2008;14:196–200.

203. Savage SA, Irani SR, Leite MI, Zeman AZ. NMDA receptor antibody encephalitis presenting as transient epileptic amnesia. J Neuroimmunol. 2019;327:41–3.
204. Cretin B, Bilger M, Philippi N, Blanc F. CASPR2 antibody encephalitis presenting as transient epileptic amnesia. Seizure. 2020;81:175–7.
205. Oagawa S, Uchida Y, Kobayashi S, Takeda K, Terada K, Matsukawa N. GABA$_B$ receptor autoimmune encephalitis presenting as transient epileptic amnesia. Rinsho Shinkeigaku. 2021;61:6–11.
206. Rojas-Marcos I, Fernandez A, Caballero JA, Suarez A, Blanco A. Familial transient epileptic amnesia. Report of three siblings. J Neurol. 2012;259(Suppl1):S178. (abstract P672)
207. Paccagnella E, Gosavi TD, Neligan A, Walker M. Transient epileptic amnesia: an unusual case report. Poster presentation, BNA/ABN Meeting of Minds symposium, Cardiff, UK, 29 September 2016.
208. Romoli M, Tuna MA, Li L, et al. Time trends, frequency, characteristics and prognosis of short-duration transient global amnesia. Eur J Neurol. 2020;27:887–93.
209. Ung KYC, Larner AJ. Transient amnesia: epileptic or global? A differential diagnosis with significant implications for management. Q J Med. 2014;107:915–7.
210. Greene HH, Bennett DR. Transient global amnesia with a previously unreported EEG abnormality. Electroencephalogr Clin Neurophysiol. 1974;36:409–13.
211. Zorzon M, Antonutti L, Mase G, Biasutti E, Vitrani B, Cazzato G. Transient global amnesia and transient ischemic attack. Natural history, vascular risk factors, and associated conditions. Stroke. 1995;26:1536–42.
212. Fouchard AA, Biberon J, Mondon K, de Toffol B. Transient epileptic amnesia secondary to hippocampal dysplasia mimicking transient global amnesia. Seizure. 2016;43:23–5.
213. Sugiyama A, Kobayashi M, Matsunaga T, Kanai T, Kuwabara S. Transient global amnesia with a hippocampal lesion followed by transient epileptic amnesia. Seizure. 2015;31:141–3.
214. Zola-Morgan S, Squire LR, Amaral DG. Human amnesia and the medial temporal region: enduring memory impairment following a bilateral lesion limited to field CA1 of the hippocampus. J Neurosci. 1986;6:2950–67.
215. Auyeung M, Tsoi TH, Cheung CM, et al. Association of diffusion weighted imaging abnormalities and recurrence in transient global amnesia. J Clin Neurosci. 2011;18:531–4.
216. Lampl Y, Sadeh M, Lorberboym M. Transient global amnesia—not always a benign process. Acta Neurol Scand. 2004;110:75–9.
217. Harrison NA, Johnston K, Corno F, et al. Psychogenic amnesia: syndromes, outcome, and patterns of retrograde amnesia. Brain. 2017;140:2498–510.
218. Kritchevsky M, Chang J, Squire LR. Functional amnesia: clinical description and neuropsychological profile of 10 cases. Learn Mem. 2004;11:213–26.
219. Pujol M, Kopelman M. Psychogenic amnesia. Pract Neurol. 2003;3:292–9.
220. Staniloiu A, Markowitsch HJ. Dissociative amnesia. Lancet Psychiatry. 2014;1:226–41.
221. Gil R, Abdul-Samad F, Mathis S, Neau JP. Was there a confusion before 1950 between global transient global [sic] amnesia and psychogenic amnesia? [in French]. Rev Neurol (Paris). 2010;166:699–703.
222. Merriam AE. Emotional arousal-induced transient global amnesia. Case report, differentiation from hysterical amnesia, and an etiologic hypothesis. Neuropsychiatry Neuropsychol Behav Neurol. 1988;1:73–8.
223. Markowitsch HJ, Staniloiu A. The impairment of recollection in functional amnesic states. Cortex. 2013;49:1494–510.
224. Baxendale S. Memories aren't made of these: amnesia at the movies. BMJ. 2004;329:1480–3.
225. Larner AJ. "Neurological literature": cognitive disorders. Adv Clin Neurosci Rehabil. 2008;8(2):20.
226. Larner AJ. Unconscious driving phenomenon. Adv Clin Neurosci Rehabil. 2011;10(6):26.
227. Moersch F. Psychic manifestations of migraine. Am J Psych. 1924;80:697–716.
228. Evans JH. Transient loss of memory, an organic mental syndrome. Brain. 1966;89:539–48.

229. Gilbert JJ, Benson DF. Transient global amnesia: report of two cases with definite etiologies. J Nerv Ment Dis. 1972;154:461–4.
230. Laplane D, Truelle JL. The mechanism of transient global amnesia. Apropos of some unusual cases [in French]. Nouv Presse Med. 1974;3:721–5.
231. Frank G. Amnestic episodes in migraine. A contribution to the differential diagnosis of transient global amnesia (ictus amnésique) [in German]. Schweiz Arch Neurol Neurochir Psychiatr. 1976;118:253–74.
232. Caplan L, Chedru F, Lhermitte F, Mayman C. Transient global amnesia and migraine. Neurology. 1981;31:1167–70.
233. Olivarius BD, Jensen TS. Transient global amnesia in migraine. Headache. 1979;19:335–8.
234. Lane R, Davies P. Migraine. New York: Taylor & Francis; 2006.
235. Haas DC, Ross GS. Transient global amnesia triggered by mild head trauma. Brain. 1986;109:251–7.
236. Pacheva I, Ivanov I. Acute confusional migraine: is it a distinct form of migraine? Int J Clin Pract. 2013;67:250–6.
237. Miller JW, Petersen RC, Metter EJ, Millikan CH, Yanagihara T. Transient global amnesia: clinical characteristics and prognosis. Neurology. 1987;37:733–7.
238. Schipper S, Riederer F, Sander PS, Gantenbein AR. Acute confusional migraine: our knowledge to date. Expert Rev Neurother. 2012;12:307–14.
239. Sheth RD, Riggs JE, Bodensteiner JB. Acute confusional migraine: variant of transient global amnesia. Pediatr Neurol. 1995;12:129–31.
240. Larner AJ. Acute confusional migraine and transient global amnesia: variants of cognitive migraine? Int J Clin Pract. 2013;67:1066.
241. Szabo K, Hoyer C, Caplan LR, et al. Diffusion-weighted MRI in transient global amnesia and its diagnostic implications. Neurology. 2020;95:e206–12.
242. Maffei D, Grizzi F, Zanoni M, Vota P, Justich M, Taverna G. Recurrent transient global amnesia after intracavernous Caverject injection in erectile dysfunction after robotic prostatectomy. Urol Case Rep. 2020;31:101184.
243. Grande LA, Loeser JD, Samil A. Recurrent transient global amnesia with intrathecal baclofen. Anesth Analg. 2008;106:1284–7.
244. Mumenthaler M, Kaeser HE, Meyer A, Hess T. Transient global amnesia after clioquinol: five personal observations from outside Japan. J Neurol Neurosurg Psychiatry. 1979;42:1084–90.
245. Kaeser HE. Transient global amnesia due to clioquinol. Acta Neurol Scand Suppl. 1984;100:175–83.
246. Mazzucchi A, Moretti G, Caffarra P, Parma M. Neuropsychological functions in the follow-up of transient global amnesia. Brain. 1980;103:161–78.
247. Otrock ZK, Beydoun A, Barada WM, Masroujeh R, Hourani R, Bazarbachi A. Transient global amnesia associated with the infusion of DMSO-cryopreserved autologous peripheral blood stem cells. Haematologica. 2008;93:e36–7.
248. Gil-Martinez T, Galiano R. Transient global amnesia following the use of ergots in the treatment of migraine [in Spanish]. Rev Neurol. 2004;39:929–31.
249. Teh CH, Robertson MN, Warkentin TE, Henriksen PA, Brackenbury ET, Anderson JA. Transient global amnesia as the presenting feature of heparin-induced thrombocytopenia. J Card Surg. 2010;25:300–2.
250. Sandyk R. Transient global amnesia induced by lorazepam. Clin Neuropharmacol. 1985;8:297–8.
251. Stracciari A, Guarino M, Crespi C, Pazzaglia P. Transient amnesia triggered by acute marijuana intoxication. Eur J Neurol. 1999;6:521–3.
252. Shukla PC, Moore UB. Marijuana-induced transient global amnesia. South Med J. 2004;97:782–4.
253. Mansour G, Abuzaid A, Bellamkonda P. I do not even remember what I smoked! A case of marijuana-induced transient global amnesia. Am J Med. 2014;127:e5–6.

254. Jones RJ, Brace SR, Vander Tuin EL. Probable propafenone-induced transient global amnesia. Ann Pharmacother. 1995;29:586–90.
255. Hirschfeld G, Sperfeld AD, Kassubek J, Scharffetter-Kochanek K, Sunderkotter C. Transient global amnesia (TGA) during an oral provocation test [in German]. Hautarzt. 2007;58:149–52.
256. Healy D, Morgan R, Chinnaswamy S. Transient global amnesia associated with statin intake. BMJ Case Rep. 2009;2009:pii: bcr06.2008.0033.
257. Fu PK, Hsu HY, Wang PY. Transient global amnesia after taking sibutramine: a case report. Neurologist. 2010;16:129–31.
258. Savitz SA, Caplan LR. Transient global amnesia after sildenafil (Viagra) use. Neurology. 2002;59:778.
259. Gandolfo C, Sugo A, Del Sette M. Sildenafil and transient global amnesia. Neurol Sci. 2003;24:145–6.
260. Shihman B, Auriel E, Bornstien NM. Two cases of transient global amnesia (TGA) following sildenafil use [in Hebrew]. Harefuah. 2006;145(656-7):703.
261. Marques-Vilallonga A, Aranda-Rodriguez S, Trallero-Araguas E, Jimenez-Moreno FX. Transient global amnesia associated to sildenafil and sexual activity [in Spanish]. Rev Neurol. 2014;59:93.
262. Finsterer J. Transient global amnesia associated with sildenafil use. Report of one case. Rev Med Chil. 2019;147:527–9.
263. Lin KY, Liu MN, Wang PH, Lau CI. Positive magnetic resonance imaging evidence of transient global amnesia following the use of sildenafil. Clin Neuropharmacol. 2020;43:52–3.
264. Lee E, Ghafoor N, Jefri M, Black AD, Calello DP, Santos CD. Acute coronary syndrome and transient global amnesia with sumatriptan. Am J Emerg Med. 2021; S0735-6757(21)00754-3. Online ahead of print
265. Schiefer J, Sparing R. Transient global amnesia after intake of tadalafil, a PDE-5 inhibitor: a possible association? Int J Impot Res. 2005;17:383–4.
266. Bardes I, Pujadas F, Ibarria M, Boada M. Transient global amnesia after tadalafil use [in Spanish]. Med Clin (Barc). 2008;131:78.
267. Machado A, Rodrigues M, Ribeiro M, Cerqueira J, Soares-Fernandes J. Tadalafil-induced transient global amnesia. J Neuropsychiatry Clin Neurosci. 2010;22:e28.
268. Morris HH 3rd, Estes ML. Traveler's [sic] amnesia. Transient global amnesia secondary to triazolam. JAMA. 1987;258:945–6.
269. Tsai MY, Tsai MH, Yang SC, Tseng YL, Chuang YC. Transient global amnesia-like episode due to mistaken intake of zolpidem: drug safety concern in the elderly. J Patient Saf. 2009;5:32–4.
270. Zeman A, Hoefeijzers S, Milton F, Dewar M, Carr M, Streatfield C. The GABAB receptor agonist, baclofen, contributes to three distinct varieties of amnesia in the human brain—a detailed case report. Cortex. 2016;74:9–19.
271. Ansseau M, Poncelet PF, Schmitz D. High dose triazolam and anterograde amnesia. BMJ. 1992;304:1178.
272. Brown J, Lewis V, Brown M, Horn G, Bowes JB. A comparison between transient amnesias induced by two drugs (diazepam or lorazepam) and amnesia of organic origin. Neuropsychologia. 1982;20:55–70.
273. Danek A, Uttner I, Straube A. Is transient global amnesia related to endogenous benzodiazepines? J Neurol. 2002;249:628.
274. Caplan LB. [sic]. Transient global amnesia. In: Frederiks JAM, editor. Handbook of clinical neurology. Volume 1 (45). Clinical neuropsychology. Amsterdam: Elsevier Science Publishers; 1985. p. 205–18.
275. Parkin AJ, Leng NRC. Neuropsychology of the amnesic syndrome. Hove: Lawrence Erlbaum Associates; 1993.
276. Durrani M, Milas J, Parson G, Pescatore R. Temporary memory steal: transient global amnesia secondary to nephrolithiasis. Clin Pract Cases Emerg Med. 2018;2:334–7.

277. Chalmers J, Risk MT, Kean DM, Grant R, Ashworth B, Campbell IW. Severe amnesia after hypoglycemia. Clinical, psychometric, and magnetic resonance imaging correlations. Diabetes Care. 1991;14:922–5.
278. Holemans X, Dupuis M, Missan N, Vanderijst J-F. Reversible amnesia in a type 1 diabetic patient and bilateral hippocampal lesions on magnetic resonance imaging (MRI). Diabet Med. 2001;18:761–3.
279. Larner AJ, Moffat MA, Ghadiali E, Majid S, English P, Williams G. Amnesia following profound hypoglycaemia in a type 1 diabetic patient. Eur J Neurol. 2003;10(Suppl1):92. (abstract P1170)
280. Cox C, Larner AJ. Recurrent hypoglycaemia and cognitive impairment: a 14-year follow-up. Br J Hosp Med. 2016;77:540–1.
281. Kirchhoff BA, Lugar HM, Smith SE, et al. Hypoglycaemia-induced changes in regional brain volume and memory function. Diabet Med. 2013;30:e151-6.
282. Koempfen M. Observation sur un cas de perte de mémoire. Mémoires de l'Academie Nationale de Médecine. 1835;4:489–94.
283. Ribot T. Diseases of memory: an essay in the positive psychology. New York: D Appleton and Company; 1882.
284. Larner AJ. Did Ribot describe transient global amnesia in the nineteenth century? Cortex. 2021;138:38–9.
285. Fisher CM. Concussion amnesia. Neurology. 1966;16:826–30.
286. Friedland D, Swash M. Post-traumatic amnesia and confusional state: hazards of retrospective assessment. J Neurol Neurosurg Psychiatry. 2016;87:1068–74.
287. Marshman LA, Jakabek D, Hennessy M, Quirk F, Guazzo EP. Post-traumatic amnesia. J Clin Neurosci. 2013;20:1475–81.
288. Ardila A. Transient global amnesia resulting from mild trauma. Neuropsychology. 1989;3:23–7.
289. Moral A, Beltran A. Transient global amnesia following slight cranial injury. Neurologia. 1988;3:124–5.
290. Vohanka S, Zouhar A. Transient global amnesia after mild head injury in childhood. Acta Nerv Super (Praha). 1988;30:68–74.
291. Accurti I, Proli F. Transient global amnesia: a personal series of idiopathic and post-traumatic cases. Ital J Neurol Sci. 1988;(Suppl 9):25–8.
292. Evans RW. The postconcussion syndrome. In: Aminoff MJ, editor. Neurology and general medicine. 4th ed. Philadelphia: Churchill Livingstone Elsevier; 2008. p. 593–603.
293. Venneri A, Brazzelli M, Della Sala S. Transient global amnesia triggered by mild head injury. Brain Inj. 1998;12:605–12.
294. Coelho P, Schön M, Alves PN, Fonseca AC, Pinho E, Melo T. An image is not always worth a thousand words: an image mimic of transient global amnesia. Neurol Sci. 2021;42:2515–7.
295. Galvin R, Brathen G, Ivashynka I, et al. EFNS guidelines for diagnosis, therapy and prevention of Wernicke encephalopathy. Eur J Neurol. 2010;17:1408–18.
296. Scalzo SJ, Bowden SC, Ambrose ML, Whelan G, Cook MJ. Wernicke-Korsakoff syndrome not related to alcohol use: a systematic review. J Neurol Neurosurg Psychiatry. 2015;86:1362–8.
297. Larner AJ, Gardner-Thorpe C. Robert Lawson (?1846-1896). J Neurol. 2012;259:792–3.
298. Sacks O. The man who mistook his wife for a hat. London: Picador; 1986.
299. Dharia S, Zeman A. Fatigue amnesia. Cortex. 2016;79:153–4.
300. American Psychiatric Association. Diagnostic and statistical manual of mental disorders. 4th ed, text revision (DSM-IV-TR). Washington: American Psychiatric Association; 2000.
301. Benon R. Les ictus amnésiques dans les démences "organiques". Ann Méd Psychol. 1909;67:207–19.
302. Benon R. Les ictus amnésiques dans la paralysie générale. Gaz Hôp (Paris). 1908;1335
303. Hall JA. Transient global amnesia in neurolues. Practitioner. 1982;226:953–5.

304. Fujimoto H, Imaizumi T, Nishimura Y, et al. Neurosyphilis showing transient global amnesia-like attacks and magnetic resonance imaging abnormalities mainly in the limbic system. Intern Med. 2001;40:439–42.
305. Kimura S, Kumano T, Miyao S, Teramoto J. Herpes simplex encephalitis with transient global amnesia as an early sign. Intern Med. 1995;34:131–3.
306. McCorry DJ, Crowley P. Transient global amnesia secondary to herpes simplex viral encephalitis. Q J Med. 2005;98:154–5.
307. Pommer B, Pilz P, Harrer G. Transient global amnesia as a manifestation of Epstein-Barr virus encephalitis. J Neurol. 1983;229:125–7.
308. Young CA, Humphrey PR, Ghadiali EJ, Klapper PE, Cleator GM. Short-term memory impairment in an alert patient as a presentation of herpes simplex encephalitis. Neurology. 1992;42:260–1.
309. Smithson E, Larner AJ. Glioblastoma multiforme masquerading as herpes simplex encephalitis. Br J Hosp Med. 2013;74:52–3.
310. Hussein HM. Transient global amnesia as a possible first manifestation of COVID-19. Neurohospitalist. 2021;11:84–6.
311. Nishizawa T, Kawakami A, Taguchi T, Osugi Y. Transient global amnesia with bilateral hippocampal lesions during the COVID-19 global outbreak. J Gen Fam Med. 2020;22:154–5.
312. Werner R, Keller M, Woehrle JC. Increased incidence of transient global amnesia during the Covid-19 crisis? Neurol Res Pract. 2020;2(1):26.

Chapter 4
Investigation of TGA (1): Neuropsychology, Neurophysiology and Other Investigations

Abstract This chapter examines the investigation of TGA, particularly the neuro-psychological and neurophysiological findings (neuroimaging is considered in Chap. 5). Investigations during the TGA episode have clarified the exact nature of the neuropsychological deficit. EEG may have a role in the differential diagnosis of TGA from transient epileptic amnesia. Clinical investigations undertaken when patients are seen some time after the event are generally normal and probably unnecessary if a definite (criteria-based) clinical diagnosis of pure TGA has been made.

Keywords TGA · Neuropsychology · Neurophysiology

The investigation of TGA may be contemplated as two different scenarios: acutely, during the episode, or interval assessment at some time after the resolution of the attack. The latter has generally been the more common situation, but in recent times the increasing development of acute neurological services, sometimes embedded within emergency room (ER) or accident and emergency (A&E) settings, has enabled acute rather than interval assessment of TGA. This has prompted a change in the way TGA patients are investigated, particularly with respect to neuroimaging (Chap. 5).

4.1 Neuropsychology

There are many different tests available for neuropsychological assessment (e.g. [1, 2]), looking at either single or multiple cognitive domains, and suitable for use in different settings (primary or secondary care, general or specialised clinic) and taking different periods of time to complete (minutes to hours). Those addressing memory function have been most relevant in TGA.

A.J. Larner, *Transient Global Amnesia*,
https://doi.org/10.1007/978-3-030-98939-2_4

Discussion here is largely restricted to definite or pure TGA as defined by the Hodges and Warlow 1990 criteria [3], with only passing reference to possible variant forms of TGA (see Sect. 2.3 for further details of these).

Reports of neuropsychological assessments undertaken during an attack of TGA are relatively uncommon. Indeed, it was not until the 1980s that detailed reports first began to appear (e.g. [4–11] and [12], p.68–78,139–44). Essentially, these showed that pure TGA is characterised by anterograde amnesia (difficulty learning new information) which is often described as severe, dense or profound since new information is lost within minutes, with in addition a retrograde amnesia (loss of previously learned information) extending over very variable time periods in different patients ranging from hours to decades, patchy but showing a temporal gradient. Other domains of cognitive function generally remain intact. Complete recovery except for permanent retrograde amnesia for events that occurred several hours to days before the TGA event is usual.

4.1.1   Neuropsychological Deficits during TGA: Memory

Memory may be conceptualised as a non-uniform, distributed cognitive function within which subdivisions in function may be differentiated (Fig. 2.2): explicit or declarative (episodic, semantic) and implicit on non-declarative. Neuropsychological assessment of each of these memory subdivisions has been undertaken during episodes of TGA.

4.1.1.1   "Working Memory"

"Working memory", or immediate memory, is usually conceptualised as one aspect of attentional mechanisms, rather than mnestic function per se, but since preserved attentional mechanisms are required for any meaningful assessment of memory function the assessment of working memory is an important first step in any neuropsychological evaluation. Acute confusional states (delirium), which enter the differential diagnosis of TGA (Sect. 3.5.1), are characterised by impaired attentional mechanisms.

Working memory is preserved in TGA, as manifested by normal performance on tests in both the verbal (normal forward and backward digit span tests) and nonverbal (block tapping span) domains (e.g. [12], p.70 and [6]).

Quinette et al. [13] examined working memory in more detail, using tests to investigate the various subcomponents in the model of working memory proposed by Baddeley [14]. They showed that the phonological loop and visuospatial sketch pad functions were spared, as were many of the specific executive functions.

4.1.1.2 Anterograde Memory

Characteristically, testing during a TGA attack has shown dense anterograde amnesia, with impairment of new learning ability for material presented either verbally or non-verbally [9, 12].

Verbal material includes recalling a story (e.g. from the Wechsler Memory Scale) or learning word lists. In addition to a low global score on the latter, there may be impairment of the primacy effect but with relative preservation of the recency effect [15].

Non-verbal material includes recall of the Rey–Osterrieth Complex Figure, copying of which is generally good (see Sect. 4.1.2.2). Hodges ([12], p.72) found that none of his subjects could reproduce any elements of the Rey–Osterrieth Complex Figure after a delay of approximately 40 min. Supraspan block tapping test is also a test of non-verbal learning; none of Hodges' patients could learn these sequences, confirming previous findings [4, 5].

Is the observed anterograde amnesia a consequence of failure to acquire, encode or store new information, or is the deficit one of retrieval? This issue may be addressed by investigating whether there is differential performance in tests of recall or recognition. To examine specifically episodic memory, Eustache et al. [16] administered a word-learning task (derived from the Grober and Buschke procedure) to three patients during episodes of TGA. In one patient, there was poor performance on immediate cued recall, a result which suggested an encoding deficit, whereas in the other two patients there was poor performance on delayed recall and recognition, suggesting a storage deficit. Whether this represented heterogeneity within cases of TGA, or different degrees of dysfunction within a common mechanism for encoding and retrieval, was not clear [16, 17], but a later study of two additional patients [18] pointed towards cognitive heterogeneity, one patient having a storage disturbance, whilst the other was unable to learn episodic associations, despite similar neurological features.

A meta-analysis of 25 studies examining the cognitive characteristics of TGA found "an extraordinarily large reduction" of anterograde memory [19].

4.1.1.3 Retrograde Memory

Retrograde amnesia in TGA is of variable duration, ranging from hours to decades, although in most patients it is less than 5 years. The deficit, although patchy, is temporally graded, affecting memory for both personal and public events ([12], p.74–8,81–5, and [6, 8, 9]).

As regards assessment of personal retrograde memory, this is recognised to be difficult to quantify. The Crovitz test of cued autobiographical memory has been reported to show that TGA patients have difficulty in producing personal memories, particularly for the most recent 5 years, and that these accounts are impoverished in terms of detail ([12], p.77–8,83–4, and [6, 9]). Impaired ability to describe detailed life episodes has also been noted using the Autobiographical Memory Interview [20].

In contrast to patients with functional amnesia (Sect. 3.3), TGA patients preferentially use the first person pronoun rather than general pronouns when recounting autobiographical narratives [21].

For assessment of public retrograde memory, various tests may be used, such as the Famous Faces Test (identifying famous people from previous decades) and famous events (dating significant previous events). Such studies indicate a temporal gradient, with poorer performance on more recent material but with more distant memories relatively spared.

A meta-analysis of 25 studies examining the cognitive characteristics of TGA found a milder reduction of retrograde compared to anterograde memory [19]. A permanent retrograde amnesia for events that occurred several hours to days before the TGA event is usual.

4.1.1.4   Semantic Memory

Semantic memory, assessed by category fluency measures, picture naming, and picture–word and picture–picture matching, and reading ability was normal during TGA in two patients assessed by Hodges [22]. More recently, however, Sandikci et al. [23] found impaired semantic fluency in 16 patients during TGA (with typical neuroimaging findings) compared to their function one day later. They suggest their findings support a role for the hippocampus in semantic retrieval.

A possible TGA variant in which transient impairment of semantic memory was present has been described ([24]; see Sect. 2.3.3).

4.1.1.5   Implicit Memory

Implicit memory functions (e.g. for driving; see Sect. 6.4.1) are usually intact in TGA [6]. Indeed, procedural memories for motor and perceptual skills can be acquired during TGA episodes [25, 26], confirming the empirical dissociability of explicit and implicit memory processes. Eustache et al. [15] examined perceptual-verbal procedural memory (mirror reading skill learning task) and lexical–semantic priming (word stem completion task) in a TGA patient and found these abilities to be preserved compared to controls despite the patient's profound explicit memory impairment. Guillery et al. [27] demonstrated semantic priming in three TGA patients, effects which persisted at least 1 day after recovery from TGA, suggesting the possibility of semantic learning without episodic memory.

A possible TGA variant in which procedural memory impairment is present has been described (Sect. 2.3.4).

4.1.1.6   Spatial Memory

Experimental animal studies have suggested that the hippocampus has a function as a cognitive map, underpinning spatial memory [28]. In the light of the focal hippocampal lesions seen on magnetic resonance imaging in TGA patients (see Sect.

5.1.2), Bartsch et al. [29] examined place learning using a virtual Morris water maze in TGA patients with hippocampal lesions. Compared to controls, TGA patients showed a profound impairment of place learning, the deficits in performance correlated with the size of hippocampal lesions and duration of TGA.

More sophisticated tests of hippocampal function have indicated selective and prolonged deficits in allocentric (hippocampus-dependent) spatial navigation in patients following TGA [30] suggesting that damage had occurred within the hippocampus.

4.1.1.7 Metamemory

The term metamemory has been used to describe knowledge about one's memory processes and contents. It has been little studied in TGA compared to other aspects of memory. Neri et al. [31] used the Sehulster Memory Scale [32] to assess metamemory in 20 patients with a previous episode of TGA, finding metamemory evaluations to be more closely related to objective memory function in those with more severe residual retrograde amnesia [31]. Imprecision of metamemory was also reported in TGA patients by Marin-Garcia and Ruiz-Vargas [33].

4.1.2 Neuropsychological Deficits during TGA: Other Cognitive Domains

Cognitive domains other than memory are typically preserved in TGA, such as language, visuospatial function [6] and frontal executive functions [13, 22].

4.1.2.1 Language

All aspects of language tested by Hodges ([12], p.79) were normal.

4.1.2.2 Visuoperceptual and Visuospatial Skills

All aspects of visuoperceptual/visuospatial function tested by Hodges ([12], p.79) were normal. However, reduced ability to copy the Rey–Osterrieth Complex Figure has been observed [8, 9], suggesting to these authors a cognitive deficit separate from and in addition to the amnesia. However, this report would seem to be exceptional.

4.1.2.3   Executive Function

Stillhard et al. [11] found reduced verbal fluency and evidence of colour–word inter-
ference in the Stroop test in their patient, suggestive of frontal lobe dysfunction.

A meta-analysis of 25 studies examining the cognitive characteristics of TGA
found diminished executive functions, suggesting that non-amnestic cognitive
changes may be found in TGA [19].

4.1.3   Neuropsychological Deficits after TGA

Comparison of mnestic function during and a few weeks after TGA usually shows
return to normal of both anterograde and retrograde memory [20]. However, testing
earlier after the acute episode, for example, after 3 or 4 days, may show persisting
impairments in verbal and non-verbal long-term memory and verbal fluency [34],
whereas testing at longer time periods may show no difference from controls (e.g.
[35, 36]). Cognitive outcomes in the post-acute and longer term following TGA are
considered in the Chapter on prognosis (Sect. 6.1 and Sect. 6.3.1, respectively).

Of the various brief ("bedside") cognitive screening instruments which are available (for discussion see [37]), a number have been used by the author in patients
who have had attacks of TGA. These have included the Mini-Mental State
Examination [38] (MMSE; see Case Study 2.1), the Six-Item Cognitive Impairment
Test [39] (6CIT), the Montreal Cognitive Assessment [40] (MoCA; see Case Study
2.1), the AD8 [41, 42], the Mini-Addenbrooke's Cognitive Examination [43]
(MACE) and Free-Cog [44] as part of pragmatic diagnostic test accuracy studies
[45, 46] of these tests [47–53]. In the majority of cases, these have returned normal
scores, the exception being two patients judged to have mild cognitive impairment
(aged 73 and 79) independent of their TGA attack (Larner, unpublished
observations).

4.2   Neurophysiology

4.2.1   Electroencephalography (EEG)

The suspicion that TGA might be an epileptic phenomenon prompted investigation
with standard electroencephalography (EEG) post-event in several of the earliest
reports (e.g. [54–57]) and this trend continued; the first report devoted to EEG in
TGA was that of Jaffe and Bender of 1966 in which 27 of 51 cases underwent EEG,
5 during the event [58].

Although most reported EEG studies were negative or showed only non-specific
changes (e.g. temporal slow waves), occasional reports of spike and wave discharges
on interictal recordings appeared, seeming to support an epileptic aetiology for
TGA (e.g. [59–62], at least in some cases. However, with hindsight some of these

patients may have had epilepsy rather than TGA, the reports predating publication of TGA diagnostic criteria [3] and characterisation of TEA. Reviews by Pedley (1983) [63], Miller et al. (1987) [64] and Jacome (1989) [65] suggested that some EEG changes reported in TGA were in fact non-specific or represented benign sleep spikes or changes seen in migraine (e.g. [66]). Nevertheless, some authors continued to hold the view that TGA is a form of epilepsy, the electrical changes being too deep for detection by surface EEG recordings (e.g. [67, 68]). Furthermore, recordings made after the TGA episode might not be reflective of the situation during attacks.

4.2.2 EEG during TGA

Reports of EEG recordings during an episode of TGA have been relatively sparse and often a consequence of chance. Generally, as for interictal studies, these have been entirely normal (e.g. [58, 64, 69, 70] and [12], p.65,141; see also Case Study 4.1), although occasional positive findings are reported: Jeong et al. [71] found bitemporal sharp waves accentuated by hyperventilation in a patient with TGA and typical diffusion-weighted magnetic resonance imaging findings (Sect. 5.1.2); EEG changes disappeared with recovery.

Case Study 4.1: EEG during TGA
A 58-year-old lady presented to her local hospital with confusion. She was unable to give a history of what had happened, but her husband reported that she had appeared distressed and was repeatedly asking the same question. She could not remember where she had been on holiday the week before or whether her mother was alive or dead. The episode settled spontaneously after about 6 h. The patient had no subsequent recollection of this period. She was otherwise in good health, with a history of only infrequent migraine. Her general and neurological examinations at presentation were normal. A provisional diagnosis of transient ischaemic attack was made by the local stroke coordinator, but the managing clinician was uncertain as to whether the episode may have been an epileptic seizure, so made arrangements for an outpatient EEG and advised the patient not to drive in the meantime.

About 10 min into the EEG recording, a further similar episode of confusion occurred: the patient was noted to be distressed, did not know where she was or how she had gotten there and repeatedly asked the same questions. The EEG coincident with this episode was normal throughout. Confusion lasted in all about 6 h, without subsequent recall. The patient later admitted to having been very anxious about attending for the EEG.

The patient was subsequently referred to the neurology clinic where, in addition to the above clinical history, collateral history from the husband elicited the fact that the first episode occurred shortly after sexual intercourse. The history was entirely consistent with diagnostic criteria for transient global amnesia (adapted from [70]).

Hence, standard EEG is of little value in the diagnosis of TGA but may have value in the differential diagnosis of attacks of TGA from TEA (Sect. 3.2, Table 2.1 and Table 3.7) if there is doubt on clinical grounds, in which case sleep-deprived EEG may increase the chances of finding changes suggestive of TEA.

More sophisticated quantitative analytic techniques evaluating EEG power spectra (qEEG) may have acute diagnostic [72] and differential diagnostic value versus TEA [73]. Comparing resting-state EEGs obtained both acutely and after recovery from TGA has been reported to show deterioration in network efficiency of the theta band frequency during the attack [74].

4.2.3   Magnetoencephalography (MEG)

Magnetoencephalography (MEG) measures magnetic fields generated by ongoing brain ionic current flows. A couple of studies examining MEG in TGA have appeared [75, 76] but neither provided significant information about underlying changes in brain activity.

4.2.4   Transcranial Magnetic Stimulation (TMS)

Nardone et al. [77] investigated one case of TGA with TMS and found decreased intracortical inhibition (ICI) during the attack.

4.3   Other Investigations

If the clinical diagnosis of "pure" TGA (Sect. 2.2.2) is made, then other investigations are generally unnecessary.

4.3.1   Blood Tests

Standard or routine tests of haematology and blood chemistry seldom, if ever, have any place in the investigation of patients with suspected or confirmed TGA. Occasional reports of abnormal blood tests in TGA have appeared, but generally they constitute anecdotal evidence only. For example, there are occasional reports of TGA occurring in patients with polycythaemia, for example, in association with polycythaemia rubra vera (PRV) [78, 79] and cerebellar haemangioblastoma [80]. In one PRV case [79], multiple recurrences were reported (which may prompt questions about the TGA diagnosis), ceasing with the treatment of polycythaemia. In the light of these cases, an argument might be made for checking indices such as haematocrit, red cell mass and blood volume and blood viscosity. However, Hodges ([12], p.132) found no significant difference in packed cell volume between TGA patients and TIA controls. Only 1 of 24 TGA patients in the series of Moreno-Lugris et al. [81] had polycythaemia.

Other markers of vascular and/or inflammatory involvement have been examined in TGA patients. For example, hyperfibrinogenaemia, a marker of inflammation, was reported in a patient who developed recurrent episodes of TGA after cardiac surgery, which were manifest only in the upright posture but which resolved promptly when supine [82]. As with other reports of frequently recurrent TGA (Sect. 6.2.1), there must be questions around the diagnosis of TGA here.

Cervera et al. [83] reported a cohort of 1000 patients with antiphospholipid antibody (Hughes') syndrome, of whom 0.7% had "transient amnesia". It has been reported that TGA (and migraine) is more common in Latin American patients with the antiphospholipid syndrome (APS+) than in European APS+ patients [84]. However, it remains to be determined if there is an aetiological relationship with TGA. If there are stigmata of specific vascular diseases (e.g. Sneddon syndrome, scleroderma; Sect. 3.1.4), then checking of relevant autoantibodies might be considered, but not as a routine.

Mazokopakis [85] reported five TGA patients with high serum total homocysteine levels, low serum folate and vitamin B12 and with underlying mutations in the methylenetetrahydrofolate reductase (MTHFR) gene. Hyperhomocysteinaemia, a recognised vascular risk factor, may thus be a risk factor for TGA in some cases. It has been recorded in other case reports ([86, 87] and [88], case1).

A case of TGA with elevation of highly sensitive troponin T levels was reported by Jalanko et al. [89]. This is usually a marker of cardiac ischaemia but may sometimes be seen in acute neurological disorders such as subarachnoid haemorrhage, stroke, TIA, epileptic seizures and traumatic head injury. Eisele et al. [90] found elevated high-sensitivity cardiac troponin I (hs-cTNI) in 17 of 202 TGA patients, but none had clinical or electrocardiographic evidence of myocardial infarction although two had Takotsubo syndrome (see Sect. 3.1.6). Those with elevated hs-cTNI had a significantly greater likelihood of a history of coronary heart disease and a significantly shorter TGA duration at presentation.

Neuron-specific enolase (NSE) may be used as a marker of neuronal cell dysfunction. Lee et al. found NSE to be elevated in 16/48 TGA patients, and these subjects had higher levels of cognitive impairment than those with normal levels [91].

Markers of endocrinological function have sometimes been examined in TGA. There are occasional reports of cases occurring in patients with thyroid dysfunction, for example, as a consequence of autoimmune thyroid disease [92]. A higher rate of thyroid disorders was reported in a retrospective study of 25 TGA patients from Taiwan [93].

Prolactin levels, sometimes used as a serum marker of epileptic seizure, are normal in TGA [94].

A more significant endocrinological marker may be serum cortisol levels in the light of the possible predisposing and precipitating role of stress in TGA (Sect 7.10 and Sect. 8.1 respectively). Schneckenburger et al. [95] compared blood cortisol levels between TGA patients sampled during or shortly after the episode and found significantly higher levels in the ictal group. The results suggested reactivity of the hypothalamic–pituitary–adrenal axis. Griebe et al. [96] found elevated levels of salivary cortisol in TGA patients compared to time-matched delay samples, suggesting enhanced cortisol secretion in TGA patients. However, neither of these studies could determine whether or not these observations were cause or effect of TGA, nor whether they might be of use in the differential diagnosis of acute transient amnesias.

4.3.2   Cerebrospinal Fluid (CSF)

Lumbar puncture for studies of cerebrospinal fluid (CSF) may be indicated if TGA is mistaken for other acute neurological conditions (Sect. 3.5), such as meningitis or encephalitis (looking for markers of infection) or subarachnoid haemorrhage (looking for xanthochromia, blood products), but if the clinical diagnosis of TGA has been made then CSF analysis is not indicated. In view of the acute nature of TGA, it might be interesting to know if markers of neuronal damage, such as the proteins 14–3-3 and s100beta (sometimes looked for in suspected cases of prion disease), are positive in TGA.

It has been reported that biological antioxidant potential (BAP) is elevated in CSF of TGA patients, suggesting that oxidative stress may play a role in the pathogenesis of TGA [97].

4.3.3   Sonography

Sonographic techniques have been used to evaluate both arterial and venous phases of the intra- and extracranial circulation, with the latter producing the most contentious results.

4.3.3.1   Arterial

Extracranial and transcranial arterial echo colour Doppler sonography was undertaken in 75 TGA patients and the same number of age- and gender-matched controls by Baracchini et al. [98]. They found no evidence of significant cervical vessel or intracranial atherosclerosis. There was no difference in resistance index values of the vertebral arteries at rest and during Valsalva manoeuvre and of pulsatility index values of the major intracranial arteries at rest and during Valsalva manoeuvre. Furthermore, no difference in any study item was found between patients assessed during or soon after the TGA episode. Jovanovic et al. [99] found no significant structural atherosclerotic changes in the cervicocranial arteries on ultrasound of 100 patients with TGA.

4.3.3.2 Venous; Internal Jugular Vein Valve Incompetence

Prompted by Lewis's influential (1998) hypothesis of TGA as a consequence of cerebral venous congestion [100] (see Sect. 9.2.2 for discussion), a number of sonographic studies appeared in the early 2000s examining internal jugular vein blood flow. These detected an increased prevalence of abnormal (retrograde) internal jugular vein blood flow due to jugular vein valve incompetence during a Valsalva manoeuvre in TGA patients compared to TIA patients and normal controls (e.g. [101–103]).

Many subsequent studies addressing this issue have been published (e.g. [99, 104–108]). A meta-analysis of seven case–control studies published in 2012 confirmed the increased incidence of internal jugular vein valve incompetence in TGA patients and also showed that recognised precipitating factors for TGA (Chap. 8) were more common in this group [109]. However, despite internal jugular vein valve incompetence, there may not necessarily be any change in intracranial venous circulation [110]. For example, Baracchini et al. [111] found no difference in blood flow velocity in the deep cerebral veins at rest or during Valsalva manoeuvre in TGA patients or controls, and intracranial venous reflux was not observed. Hence, the relevance of internal jugular vein valve incompetence to the pathogenesis of TGA remains uncertain [112]. Higher rates of compression/stenosis of internal jugular veins and left brachiocephalic vein with transverse sinus hypoplasia have also been recorded in TGA patients [113].

Pragmatically, there seems little indication for undertaking such studies as a routine investigation in patients with single episode pure TGA.

4.4 Summary and Recommendations

TGA is a clinical diagnosis, even when based on widely accepted diagnostic criteria [3]. If a confident clinical diagnosis of pure TGA, based on diagnostic criteria, can be made, then no further investigation may be required (certainly none are mandatory), and management should focus on reassurance.

However, if there is diagnostic uncertainty, for example, if a compelling informant history is not available, then investigations may be required to explore and refine the differential diagnosis. Of these investigations, the precise pattern of neuropsychological deficits may be helpful, although services for acute neuropsychological assessment are not widely available. EEG may be considered if the differential diagnosis with TEA cannot be resolved on clinical grounds. Blood tests currently have little diagnostic value, although recent investigations of elevated cortisol and troponin raise the possibility that they might be of use.

Overall, the various investigational modalities considered in this chapter have little to recommend them in the acute setting. However, neuroimaging, specifically diffusion-weighted magnetic resonance imaging, has found a place. This, along with other neuroimaging techniques, is considered in the next chapter.

References

1. Lezak MD, Howieson DB, Bigler ED, Tranel D. Neuropsychological assessment. 5th ed. New York: Oxford University Press; 2012.
2. Tate RL. A compendium of tests, scales, and questionnaires. The practitioner's guide to measuring outcomes after acquired brain impairment. Hove: Psychology Press; 2010.
3. Hodges JR, Warlow CP. Syndromes of transient amnesia: towards a classification. A study of 153 cases. J Neurol Neurosurg Psychiatry. 1990;53:834–43.
4. Caffarra P, Moretti G, Mazzucchi A, Parma M. Neuropsychological testing during a transient global amnesia episode and its follow-up. Acta Neurol Scand. 1981;63:44–50.
5. Gallassi R, Lorusso S, Stracciari A. Neuropsychological findings during a transient global amnesia attack and its follow-up. Ital J Neurol Sci. 1986;7:45–9.
6. Hodges JR, Ward CD. Observations during transient global amnesia. A behavioural and neuropsychological study of five cases. Brain. 1989;112:595–620.
7. Kritchevsky M. Transient global amnesia. In: Squire LR, Butters N, editors. Neuropsychology of memory. 2nd ed. New York: Guilford Press; 1992. p. 147–55.
8. Kritchevsky M, Squire LR. Transient global amnesia: evidence for extensive temporally graded retrograde amnesia. Neurology. 1989;39:213–8.
9. Kritchevsky M, Squire LR, Zouzounis JA. Transient global amnesia: characterization of anterograde and retrograde amnesia. Neurology. 1988;38:213–9.
10. Regard M, Landis T. Transient global amnesia: neuropsychological dysfunction during attack and recovery in two "pure" cases. J Neurol Neurosurg Psychiatry. 1984;47:668–72.
11. Stillhard G, Landis T, Schiess R, Regard M, Sialer G. Bitemporal hypoperfusion in transient global amnesia: 99m-Tc-HM-PAO SPECT and neuropsychological findings during and after an attack. J Neurol Neurosurg Psychiatry. 1990;53:339–42.
12. Hodges JR. Transient amnesia. Clinical and neuropsychological aspects. London: WB Saunders; 1991.
13. Quinette P, Guillery B, Desgranges B, de la Sayette V, Viader F, Eustache F. Working memory and executive functions in transient global amnesia. Brain. 2003;126:1917–34.
14. Baddeley AD. Working memory. Oxford: Oxford University Press; 1986.
15. Eustache F, Desgranges B, Petit-Taboué MC, et al. Transient global amnesia: implicit/explicit memory dissociation and PET assessment of brain perfusion and oxygen metabolism in the acute stage. J Neurol Neurosurg Psychiatry. 1997;63:357–67.
16. Eustache F, Desgranges B, Laville P, et al. Episodic memory in transient global amnesia: encoding, storage, or retrieval deficit? J Neurol Neurosurg Psychiatry. 1999;66:148–54.
17. Zeman AZ. Episodic memory in transient global amnesia. J Neurol Neurosurg Psychiatry. 1999;66:135.
18. Guillery B, Desgranges B, de la Sayette V, Landeau B, Eustache F, Baron JC. Transient global amnesia: concomitant episodic memory and positron emission tomography assessment in two additional patients. Neurosci Lett. 2002;325:62–6.

19. Jäger T, Bazner H, Kliegel M, Szabo K, Hennerici MG. The transience and nature of cognitive impairments in transient global amnesia: a meta-analysis. J Clin Exp Neuropsychol. 2009;31:8–19.
20. Evans J, Wilson B, Wraight EP, Hodges JR. Neuropsychological and SPECT scan findings during and after transient global amnesia: evidence for the differential impairment of remote episodic memory. J Neurol Neurosurg Psychiatry. 1993;56:1227–30.
21. Becquet C, Cogez J, Dayan J, et al. Episodic autobiographical memory impairment and differences in pronoun use: study of self-awareness in functional amnesia and transient global amnesia. Front Psychol. 2021;12:624010.
22. Hodges JR. Semantic memory and frontal executive function during transient global amnesia. J Neurol Neurosurg Psychiatry. 1994;57:605–8.
23. Sandikci V, Ebert A, Hoyer C, Platten M, Szabo K. Impaired semantic memory during acute transient global amnesia. J Neuropsychol. 2022;16:149–60.
24. Hodges JR. Transient semantic amnesia: a new syndrome? J Neurol Neurosurg Psychiatry. 1997;63:548–9.
25. Kapur N, Abbott P, Footitt D, Millar J. Long-term perceptual priming in transient global amnesia. Brain Cogn. 1996;31:63–74.
26. Marin-Garcia E, Ruiz-Vargas JM, Kapur N. Mere exposure effect can be elicited in transient global amnesia. J Clin Exp Neuropsychol. 2013;35:1007–14.
27. Guillery B, Desgranges B, Katis S, de la Sayette V, Viader F, Eustache F. Semantic acquisition without memories: evidence from transient global amnesia. Neuroreport. 2001;12:3865–9.
28. O'Keefe J, Nadel L. The hippocampus as a cognitive map. Oxford: Oxford University Press; 1978.
29. Bartsch T, Schonfeld R, Muller FJ, et al. Focal lesions of human hippocampal CA1 neurons in transient global amnesia impair place memory. Science. 2010;328:1412–5.
30. Schöberl F, Irving S, Pradhan C, et al. Prolonged allocentric navigation deficits indicate hippocampal damage in TGA. Neurology. 2019;92:e234–43.
31. Neri M, Andermarcher E, De Vreese LP, Rubichi S, Sacchet C, Cipolli C. Transient global amnesia: memory and metamemory. Aging (Milano). 1995;7:423–9.
32. Schulster JR. Structure and pragmatics of a self-theory of memory. Mem Cogn. 1981;9:263–76.
33. Marin-Garcia E, Ruiz-Vargas JM. Memory and metamemory during transient global amnesia: a comparative study about long-term follow up [in Spanish]. Rev Neurol. 2011;53:15–21.
34. Kessler J, Markowitsch HJ, Rudolf J, Heiss WD. Continuing cognitive impairment after isolated transient global amnesia. Int J Neurosci. 2001;106:159–68.
35. Uttner I, Weber S, Freund W, Schmitz B, Ramspott M, Huber R. Transient global amnesia – full recovery without persistent cognitive impairment. Eur Neurol. 2007;58:146–51.
36. Uttner I, Prexl S, Freund W, Unrath A, Bengel D, Huber R. Long-term outcome in transient global amnesia patients with and without focal hyperintensities in the CA1 region of the hippocampus. Eur Neurol. 2012;67:155–60.
37. Larner AJ, editor. Cognitive screening instruments. A practical approach. 2nd ed. London: Springer; 2017.
38. Folstein MF, Folstein SE, McHugh PR. "Mini-Mental State." a practical method for grading the cognitive state of patients for the clinician. J Psychiatr Res. 1975;12:189–98.
39. Brooke P, Bullock R. Validation of a 6 item cognitive impairment test with a view to primary care usage. Int J Geriatr Psychiatry. 1999;14:936–40.
40. Nasreddine ZS, Phillips NA, Bédirian V, et al. The Montreal Cognitive Assessment, MoCA: a brief screening tool for mild cognitive impairment. J Am Geriatr Soc. 2005;53:695–9.
41. Galvin JE, Roe CM, Powlishta KK, et al. The AD8. A brief informant interview to detect dementia. Neurology. 2005;65:559–64.
42. Galvin JE, Roe CM, Xiong C, Morris JE. Validity and reliability of the AD8 informant interview in dementia. Neurology. 2006;67:1942–8.
43. Hsieh S, McGrory S, Leslie F, et al. The Mini-Addenbrooke's Cognitive Examination: a new assessment tool for dementia. Dement Geriatr Cogn Disord. 2015;39:1–11.

44. Burns A, Harrison JR, Symonds C, Morris J. A novel hybrid scale for the assessment of cognitive and executive function: the Free-Cog. Int J Geriatr Psychiatry. 2021;36:566–72.
45. Larner AJ. Dementia in clinical practice: a neurological perspective. Pragmatic studies in the cognitive function clinic. 3rd ed. London: Springer; 2018.
46. Larner AJ. Diagnostic test accuracy studies in dementia. A pragmatic approach. 2nd ed. London: Springer; 2019.
47. Abdel-Aziz K, Larner AJ. Six-item Cognitive Impairment Test (6CIT): pragmatic diagnostic accuracy study for dementia and MCI. Int Psychogeriatr. 2015;27:991–7.
48. Larner AJ. Mini-Addenbrooke's Cognitive Examination: a pragmatic diagnostic accuracy study. Int J Geriatr Psychiatry. 2015;30:547–8.
49. Larner AJ. Implications of changing the Six-item Cognitive Impairment Test cutoff. Int J Geriatr Psychiatry. 2015;30:778–9.
50. Larner AJ. AD8 informant questionnaire for cognitive impairment: pragmatic diagnostic test accuracy study. J Geriatr Psychiatry Neurol. 2015;28:198–202.
51. Larner AJ. Mini-Addenbrooke's Cognitive Examination diagnostic accuracy for dementia: reproducibility study. Int J Geriatr Psychiatry. 2015;30:1103–4.
52. Larner AJ. M-ACE vs. MoCA. A weighted comparison. Int J Geriatr Psychiatry. 2016;31:1089–90.
53. Larner AJ. Free-Cog: pragmatic test accuracy study and comparison with Mini-Addenbrooke's Cognitive Examination. Dement Geriatr Cogn Disord. 2019;47:254–63.
54. Fisher CM, Adams RD. Transient global amnesia. Trans Am Neurol Assoc. 1958;83:143–6.
55. Bender MB. Single episode of confusion with amnesia. Bull NY Acad Med. 1960;36:197–207.
56. Poser CM, Ziegler DK. Temporary amnesia as a manifestation of cerebrovascular insufficiency. Trans Am Neurol Assoc. 1960;85:221–3.
57. Fisher CM, Adams RD. Transient global amnesia. Acta Neurol Scand. 1964;40(Suppl9):1–81.
58. Jaffe R, Bender MB. E.E.G. studies in the syndrome of isolated episodes of confusion with amnesia "transient global amnesia". J Neurol Neurosurg Psychiatry. 1966;29:472–4.
59. Dugan TM, Nordgren RE, O'Leary P. Transient global amnesia associated with bradycardia and temporal lobe spikes. Cortex. 1981;17:633–7.
60. Greene HH, Bennett DR. Transient global amnesia with a previously unreported EEG abnormality. Electroencephalogr Clin Neurophysiol. 1974;36:409–13.
61. Lou H. Repeated episodes of transient global amnesia. Acta Neurol Scand. 1968;44:612–8.
62. Tharp BR. The electroencephalogram in transient global amnesia. Electroencephalogr Clin Neurophysiol. 1969;26:96–9.
63. Pedley TA. Differential diagnosis of episodic symptoms. Epilepsia. 1983;24(Suppl1):S31–44.
64. Miller JW, Yanagihara T, Petersen RC, Klass DW. Transient global amnesia and epilepsy. Electroencephalographic distinction. Arch Neurol. 1987;44:629–33.
65. Jacome DE. EEG features in transient global amnesia. Clin Electroencephalogr. 1989;20:183–92.
66. Dupuis MM, Pierre PH, Gonsette RE. Transient global amnesia and migraine in twin sisters. J Neurol Neurosurg Psychiatry. 1987;50:816–7.
67. Fisher CM. Transient global amnesia. Precipitating activities and other observations. Arch Neurol. 1982;39:605–8.
68. Tharp BR. Transient global amnesia: manifestation of medial temporal lobe epilepsy. Clin Electroencephalogr. 1979;10:54–6.
69. Cole AJ, Gloor P, Kaplan R. Transient global amnesia: the electroencephalogram at onset. Ann Neurol. 1987;22:771–2.
70. Ung KYC, Larner AJ. Transient amnesia: epileptic or global? A differential diagnosis with significant implications for management. Q J Med. 2014;107:915–7.
71. Jeong HS, Moon JS, Baek IC, Lee AY, Kim JM. Transient global amnesia with post-hyperventilation temporal sharp waves—a case report. Seizure. 2010;19:609–11.
72. Imperatori C, Farina B, Todini F, et al. Abnormal EEG power spectra in acute transient global amnesia: a quantitative EEG study. Clin EEG Neurosci. 2019;50:188–95.

73. Lanzone J, Imperatori C, Assenza G, et al. Power spectral differences between transient epileptic and global amnesia: an eLORETA quantitative EEG study. Brain Sci. 2020;10:613.
74. Park YH, Kim JY, Yi S, et al. Transient global amnesia deteriorates the network efficiency of the theta band. PLoS One. 2016;11:e0164884.
75. Mizuno-Matsumoto Y, Ishijima M, Shinosaki K, et al. Transient global amnesia (TGA) in an [sic] MEG study. Brain Topogr. 2001;13:269–74.
76. Stippich C, Kassubek J, Kober H, Soros P, Vieth JB. Time course of focal slow wave activity in transient ischemic attacks and transient global amnesia as measured by magnetoencephalography. Neuroreport. 2000;11:3309–13.
77. Nardone R, Buffone EC, Matullo MF, Tezzon F. Motor cortex excitability in transient global amnesia. J Neurol. 2004;251:42–6.
78. Matias-Guiu J, Masague I, Codina A. Transient global amnesia and high haematocrit levels. J Neurol. 1985;232:383–4.
79. Shuping JR, Rollinson RD, Toole JF. Transient global amnesia. Ann Neurol. 1980;7:281–5.
80. Toledo M, Pujadas F, Purroy F, Alvarez-Sabin J. Polycythaemia as a ready factor of transitory global amnesia [in Spanish]. Neurologia. 2005;20:317–20.
81. Moreno-Lugris XC, Martinez-Alvarez J, Branas F, Martinez-Vazquez F, Cortes-Laino JA. Transient global amnesia. Case-control study of 24 cases [in Spanish]. Rev Neurol. 1996;24:554–7.
82. Sealove BA, Aledort LM, Stacy CB, Halperin JL. Recurrent orthostatic global amnesia in a patient with postoperative hyperfibrinogenemia. J Stroke Cerebrovasc Dis. 2008;17:241–3.
83. Cervera R, Piette JC, Font J, et al. Antiphospholipid syndrome: clinical and immunologic manifestations and patterns of disease expression in a cohort of 1,000 patients. Arthritis Rheum. 2002;46:1019–27.
84. Garcia-Carrasco M, Galarza C, Gomez-Ponce M, et al. Antiphospholipid syndrome in Latin American patients: clinical and immunologic characteristics and comparison with European patients. Lupus. 2007;16:366–73.
85. Mazokopakis EE. Transient global amnesia. Have you considered hyperhomocysteinaemia? Arq Neuropsiquiatr. 2019;77:756–7.
86. Khan R, Hossain M, Nai Q, Yousif AM, Sen S. Hyperhomocysteinaemia association with transient global amnesia: a rare case report. N Am J Med Sci. 2015;7:374–6.
87. Semmler A, Klein A, Moskau S, Linnebank M. Transient global amnesia-like episode in a patient with severe hyperhomocysteinaemia. Eur J Neurol. 2007;14:e5–6.
88. Portaro S, Naro A, Cimino V, et al. Risk factors of transient global amnesia: three case reports. Medicine (Baltimore). 2018;97:e12723.
89. Jalanko M, Forsström F, Lassus J. Cardiac troponin T elevation associated with transient global amnesia: another differential diagnosis of "troponosis". Eur Heart J Acute Cardiovasc Care. 2015;4:561–4.
90. Eisele P, Baumann S, Noor L, et al. Interaction between the heart and the brain in transient global amnesia. J Neurol. 2019;266:3048–57.
91. Lee DA, Jun KR, Kim HC, Park BS, Park KM. Significance of serum neuron-specific enolase in transient global amnesia. J Clin Neurosci. 2021;89:15–9.
92. Jacobs A, Root J, Van Gorp W. Isolated global amnesia with autoimmune thyroid disease. Neurology. 2006;66:605.
93. Pai MC, Yang SS. Transient global amnesia: a retrospective study of 25 patients. Zhonghua Yi Xue Za Zhi (Taipei). 1999;62:140–5.
94. Matias-Guiu J, Garcia C, Galdos L, Codina A. Prolactin concentrations in serum unchanged in transient global amnesia. Clin Chem. 1985;31:1764.
95. Schneckenburger R, Hainselin M, Viader F, Eustache F, Quinette P. Serum cortisol levels in patients with a transient global amnesia. Rev Neurol (Paris). 2020;176:285–8.
96. Griebe M, Ebert A, Nees F, Katic K, Gerber B, Szabo K. Enhanced cortisol secretion in acute transient global amnesia. Psychoneuroendocrinology. 2019;99:72–9.

97. Kawai T, Sakakibara R, Aiba Y, Tateno F, Ogata T, Sawai S. Increased biological anti-oxidant potential in the cerebrospinal fluid of transient global amnesia patients. Sci Rep. 2021;11(1):15861.
98. Baracchini C, Farina F, Ballotta E, Meneghetti G, Manara R. No signs of intracranial arterial vasoconstriction in transient global amnesia. J Neuroimaging. 2015;25:92–6.
99. Jovanovic ZB, Pavlovic AM, Vujisic Tesic BP, et al. Comprehensive ultrasound assessment of the craniocervical circulation in transient global amnesia. J Ultrasound Med. 2018;37:479–86.
100. Lewis SL. Aetiology of transient global amnesia. Lancet. 1998;352:397–9.
101. Akkawi NM, Agosti C, Rozzini L, Anzola GP, Padovani A. Transient global amnesia and disturbance of venous flow patterns. Lancet. 2001;357:957.
102. Maalikjy Akkawi N, Agosti C, Anzola GP, et al. Transient global amnesia: a clinical and sonographic study. Eur Neurol. 2003;49:67–71.
103. Sander D, Winbeck K, Etgen T, Knapp R, Klingelhofer J, Conrad B. Disturbance of venous flow patterns in patients with transient global amnesia. Lancet. 2000;356:1982–4.
104. Agosti C, Borroni B, Akkawi N, Padovani A. Cerebrovascular risk factors and triggers in transient global amnesia patients with and without jugular valve incompetence: results from a sample of 243 patients. Eur Neurol. 2010;63:291–4.
105. Cejas C, Cisneros LF, Lagos R, Zuk C, Ameriso SF. Internal jugular vein valve incompetence is highly prevalent in transient global amnesia. Stroke. 2010;41:67–71.
106. Himeno T, Kuriyama M, Takemaru M, et al. Vascular risk factors and internal jugular venous flow in transient global amnesia: a study of 165 Japanese patients. J Stroke Cerebrovasc Dis. 2017;26:2272–8.
107. Nedelmann M, Eicke BM, Dieterich M. Increased incidence of jugular valve insufficiency in patients with transient global amnesia. J Neurol. 2005;252:1482–6.
108. Schreiber SJ, Doepp F, Klingebiel R, Valdueza JM. Internal jugular vein valve incompetence and intracranial venous anatomy in transient global amnesia. J Neurol Neurosurg Psychiatry. 2005;76:509–13.
109. Modabbernia A, Taslimi S, Ashrafi M, Modabbernia MJ, Hu HH. Internal jugular vein reflux in patients with transient global amnesia: a meta-analysis of case-control studies. Acta Neurol Belg. 2012;112:237–44.
110. Lochner P, Nedelmann M, Kaps M, Stolz E. Jugular valve incompetence in transient global amnesia. A problem revisited. J Neuroimaging. 2014;24:479–83.
111. Baracchini C, Tonello S, Farina F, et al. Jugular veins in transient global amnesia: innocent bystanders. Stroke. 2012;43:2289–92.
112. Caplan LR. Transient global amnesia and jugular vein incompetence. Stroke. 2010;41:e568.
113. Han K, Chao AC, Chang FC, et al. Obstruction of venous drainage linked to transient global amnesia. PLoS One. 2015;10(7):e0132893.

Chapter 5
Investigation of TGA (2): Neuroimaging

Abstract This chapter examines the investigation of TGA using neuroimaging techniques, (neuropsychological and neurophysiological investigations are considered in Chap. 4). Diffusion-weighted magnetic resonance imaging may show focal areas of signal change within the hippocampus, often in the CA1 subfield, in the first few days after the TGA episode. These changes may contribute to the diagnosis of TGA, although they are not currently included in diagnostic criteria and their pathogenesis remains uncertain. More sophisticated neuroimaging techniques may contribute to further understanding of the pathophysiology of TGA.

Keywords TGA · Neuroimaging

The investigation of TGA may be contemplated as two different scenarios: the more common occurrence is when the patient presents to medical attention at some time after the resolution of the attack of TGA and the much less common situation when the patient is seen during the attack itself. If a confident clinical diagnosis of pure TGA, based on diagnostic criteria, can be made, then no further investigation may be required, and management should then focus on reassurance.

Of the various investigations available, many different neuroimaging modalities, both structural and functional, have been applied to patients with TGA, including X-ray computed tomography (CT), magnetic resonance (MR) imaging, single-photon emission computed tomography (SPECT) and positron emission tomography (PET). Of these, diffusion-weighted magnetic resonance imaging has proved to be the most diagnostically informative, often showing transient abnormalities confined to the hippocampus.

5.1   Structural Neuroimaging

5.1.1   Computed Tomography (CT)

Historically, computed tomography (CT) was the first neuroimaging modality to be widely used in TGA, beginning in the 1970s and 1980s (note that prior to this time the term "brain scanning" often referred to isotope scans, for example, using technetium pertechnetate [1]).

Although some early studies reported a high prevalence of CT abnormalities, including infarction in specific vascular territories, these series may have been contaminated by non-TGA cases, prior to the definition of diagnostic criteria in 1990 [2]. In his review published in 1985, Caplan reviewed the reported CT changes in TGA and concluded that there were insufficient data to reach general conclusions [3]. Hodges and Warlow detected small deep white matter and basal ganglia lacunar infarcts and periventricular lucencies in around 10% of their cases, but these changes were thought to be incidental, since they did not involve memory eloquent brain structures [2]. Hence, in his monograph, Hodges concluded that CT scanning in TGA was nearly always normal ([4], p.31).

Various CT lesions have been reported on occasion in TGA patients, including cerebrovascular disease (infarction, haemorrhage; Tables 3.4 and 3.5) and mass lesions (Table 7.4). Although in some cases these might be instances of "symptomatic TGA" (Sect. 2.2.2 and 2.2.3), more likely the changes seen are incidental to TGA, albeit they may have implications for patient management independent of the TGA episode.

5.1.2   Magnetic Resonance (MR) Imaging

The increased resolution of magnetic resonance (MR) imaging compared to CT might have been anticipated to generate many more neuroimaging findings in TGA cases (including incidental changes, as in other MR imaging applications in neurology [5]). Although some negative studies were reported initially (e.g. [6, 7]), the particular value of diffusion-weighted imaging MR sequences (MR-DWI) soon became apparent, showing focal areas of high signal, or hyperintensity, within the medial temporal lobe and specifically within the hippocampal formation (e.g. [8–24]). Several large series of TGA patients examined with MR-DWI have subsequently been reported (e.g. [25–30]), and, at time of writing, one systematic review and meta-analysis has been presented including 22 original articles with 1732 participants [31], plus one other systematic review [32].

These studies have established MR-DWI as the neuroimaging modality of choice, if available and required, in TGA diagnosis (Fig. 5.1). A number of conclusions may be drawn from these various studies with respect to issues such as clinical phenotype, lesion location and size, and optimal timing and technical MR imaging factors.

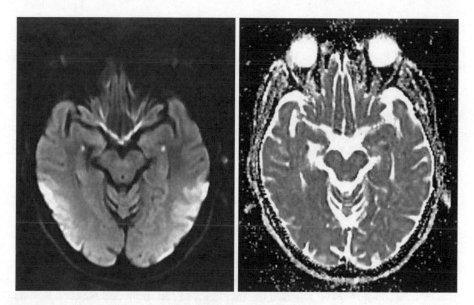

Fig. 5.1 MR brain imaging in TGA: diffusion-weighted imaging (left) and apparent diffusion coefficient map (right), 48 h after onset of TGA, showing respectively bilateral medial temporal lobe high signal and restricted diffusion (adapted from [22] with permission)

5.1.2.1   Clinical Phenotype Vs. MR-DWI Changes

TGA patients with MR-DWI lesions (DWI+) have been reported to show similar clinical characteristics to those without imaging changes (DWI−), with no significant differences in age, sex, vascular risk factors, precipitating factors or clinical presentation between the DWI+ and DWI− groups [25, 26, 33].

A small study ($n = 27$) found that patients with recurrent (i.e. a second attack of) TGA had a significantly higher association with reversible MR-DWI abnormality [34] (see Sect. 6.2.2).

5.1.2.2   Lesion Location, Number and Size

Bartsch et al. reported that most MR-DWI lesions in TGA patients were found in the CA1 (or Sommer) sector of the hippocampus (following the nomenclature of hippocampal anatomy derived from Rafael Lorente de Nó [35]), changes which gradually resolved between 3 and 10 days post-event [10, 11]. Lee et al. noted that MR-DWI lesions associated with TGA were localised exclusively to the lateral portion of the hippocampus, corresponding to the CA1 region [36]. Other studies also found the majority of TGA patients showed typical MR-DWI lesions in the CA1 region [37, 38]. However, hippocampal regions other than CA1 may be involved. For example, Kim et al. found that 23, 36 and 8 patients (= 29%, 47% and 10%) exhibited a single lesion in the hippocampal head, body and tail, respectively [27].

The systematic review of Lim et al. found figures of 12.6%, 64.4% and 23% for head, body and tail, respectively [31].

Whilst it may be the case that "[t]ypically lesions outside CA1 or outside the hippocampus are not detected in TGA" ([39], p.746), extrahippocampal hyperintense lesions have also been described in association with the typical TGA clinical phenotype on occasion [40], for example, in the splenium of the corpus callosum [9] or the cerebellum (junction of superior cerebellum and vermis) [41]. Ganeshan et al. found acute MR-DWI lesions in cortical regions other than the hippocampus in 11% of their series of TGA patients (n = 126), all presenting with typical TGA without any additional symptoms [42]. In a case series and literature review, Piffer et al. reported 26 patients with typical clinical TGA and extrahippocampal punctate diffuse lesions on MR imaging. These extrahippocampal lesions may occur with or without the typical hippocampal lesions. A classification taking these changes into account has been suggested [43]. It is possible that some of the "TGA–stroke" patients previously reported (Table 3.4) in fact have acute extrahippocampal lesions, indicative of acute focal metabolic stress but not necessarily of ischaemic origin.

Hippocampal lesions are usually single but may be multiple and may be unilateral or bilateral. Lim et al. reported the incidence of left, right and bilateral lesions to be 42%, 37% and 25%, respectively [31]. Lesion size ranged from 1 to 15.1 mm, mean 2.8–10.2 mm [31].

5.1.2.3   Timing of MR-DWI Changes

Higher MR-DWI lesion detection rates occurring after rather than during the hyperacute event have been noted by many authors (e.g. [19, 21]). Ahn et al. performed MR-DWI in 203 TGA episodes and found hippocampal lesions (= DWI+) in 16. The median time interval from amnesia to imaging was significantly longer in the DWI+ group (9 h) than in the DWI- group (5 h), indicating that MR-DWI had a low diagnostic yield (this term was not defined in the text, hence is presumably used qualitatively) if performed early in the course of TGA [25]. Ryoo et al. found an increase in the lesion detection rate with time lapse after symptom onset (0–6 h: 34%; 6–12 h: 62%; 12–24 h: 67%; day 3: 75%) [28]. Higashida et al. found that detection rate increased linearly 24 h after onset, reached a plateau by 84 h and then decreased rapidly [26]. These findings were confirmed in the systematic review by Lim et al. [31] who reported a higher diagnostic yield when DWI was performed between 24 and 96 h after symptom onset than before 24 h or after 96 h.

These data may therefore explain in part the negative findings of some of the early MR studies: Gass et al. performed DWI in the active phase in two patients and 1–8 h after cessation of symptoms in six patients [6], whilst in the series of Huber the average imaging delay was 18 h [7].

Lesions gradually resolve and disappear between 3 and 10 days post-event [10, 11, 44]. Follow-up MR imaging studies of TGA using very high field strength (7 T) showed no visible sequelae [45].

5.1.2.4   MR Field Strength, Slice Thickness and T_2-Weighting

Higher lesion detection rates have been noted in some studies dependent upon certain technical MR imaging factors, such as the use of higher MR field strength [28, 46], thinner slice thickness [29, 47] and higher resolution imaging [47]. Lim et al., in their systematic review, found no difference in diagnostic yield using 3 T vs 1.5 T field strength but higher yield using slice thickness $\leq$3 mm vs. >3 mm [31]. Considering the size range of punctate lesions, down to 1 mm and with a mean of 2.8 mm in some studies (Sect. 5.1.2.2), then clearly slice thickness of >3 mm could miss these changes. No added benefit was observed using T_2-weighted MR imaging [31] (see also Sect. 5.1.2.7).

5.1.2.5   Diagnostic Value of MR-DWI Changes

Lim et al. calculated the diagnostic yield of MR imaging as the ratio of the number of patients with small hyperintense MR-DWI lesions suggestive of TGA to the total number of patients with TGA [31], a ratio which equates to test sensitivity (i.e. ratio of true positives to sum of true positives and false negatives [48]). The pooled diagnostic yield thus defined was 39%, although there was marked heterogeneity between studies included in this systematic review (range 0–92%). Whilst this overall sensitivity is low, suggesting that there are many false negatives, yield may be improved by factors such as optimal timing of imaging (24–96 h post-TGA) and MR slice thickness ($\leq$3 mm) [31].

Wong et al. attempted to quantitate the sensitivity of MR-DWI in TGA as a function of time from symptom onset by means of a systematic review encompassing 23 papers and 1688 patients. Pooled sensitivity was reported to be 15.6% between 0 and 12 h from symptom onset, 23.1% at 0–24 h, 72.8% at 12–24 h, 68.8% at 24–36 h, 72.4% at 36–48 h, 82.8% at 46–60 h, 66.9% at 60–72 h and 72.0% at 72–96 h [32].

Dot-like hippocampal lesions, including punctate CA1 hippocampal hyperintensities, may be seen in other clinical circumstances, such as ischaemia, encephalitis, status epilepticus [49, 50], acute headache (with features different from migraine) [51] and even incidentally [52]. Förster et al. claimed that it is not possible on neuroimaging grounds alone to differentiate isolated hippocampal infarction from TGA [50]. Hence, any suggestion that MR-DWI changes are specific to TGA is incorrect, in that false-positive instances are possible, which will reduce specificity (and positive predictive value, since false-positives feature in the denominators of both these metrics [48].) The current evidence suggests that CA1 lesions are neither necessary nor sufficient for a diagnosis of TGA.

To my knowledge, a dedicated diagnostic test accuracy study of MR-DWI changes in TGA has yet to be reported. Such a study would ideally, as per other pragmatic diagnostic test accuracy studies in cognitive disorders [53], have to image all patients presenting with suspected TGA according to a predetermined imaging protocol, with diagnosis of TGA made on clinical (criterial) grounds, blind to the neuroimaging findings. Such a study would likely include patients with other conditions falling within the differential diagnosis of TGA (Chap. 3). Meantime, pending such a study or studies, the recommendation that MR-DWI may be used in the appropriate clinical setting to support the diagnosis of TGA [30] stands, allowing for the possibility of both false-negative and false-positive findings on neuroimaging. (The current widely used diagnostic criteria for TGA are exclusively clinical and do not require imaging findings [2]; Sect. 2.2.2).

5.1.2.6 Pathogenesis of MR-DWI Changes

What is the pathogenesis of the punctate lesions seen on MR-DWI in TGA patients? Many early studies interpreted the appearances as indicative of ischaemia (e.g. [10, 11, 15, 23]), but their time course is not that of a classic ischaemic lesion nor do they resemble venous congestion or infarcts.

As discussed (Sect. 5.1.2.5), the typical MR-DWI appearances seen in TGA are not specific for ischaemia, although very occasional cases of acute stroke may mimic the phenotype of TGA (Sect. 3.1.2; Table 3.4). Certainly, the CA1 region of the hippocampus is known to be particularly vulnerable to hypoxia and selective injury may be associated with amnesia (e.g. [54–56]). Other investigational modalities (MRS; Sect. 5.2.4) suggest that some form of acute metabolic stress occurs [57], but the exact pathogenesis currently remains uncertain (see Sect. 9.7.5 and 9.7.6 for further discussion).

Although finding MR-DWI changes may be helpful in differential diagnosis (Chap. 3) in the appropriate clinical circumstances [30], the suggestion that these changes indicate that TGA is a disease process localised or in some way restricted to CA1 may be challenged, both empirically and conceptually. Empirically, CA1 lesions may not be seen in some TGA cases, and extrahippocampal lesions without CA1 involvement may occur (Sect. 5.1.2.2); moreover, the imaging changes become increasingly apparent with time after the clinical event (Sect. 5.1.2.3) suggesting they are downstream events. Conceptually, damage to a specific area associated with a specific functional consequence does not necessarily indicate that that particular location is responsible for that particular function. Whilst the method of lesion observation may assist in clinico-anatomical or clinico-radiological correlation, the observed lesion may have simply interrupted fibres of passage, abolished tonic "permissive" inputs or interfered with blood supply to tissue elsewhere (transient diaschisis) ([58], p.15–16).

Thus, to describe TGA as a "natural lesion model of hippocampal CA1 neurons" ([39], p.737) appears to be an oversimplification, and data interpretation which "critically relies on the selectivity of CA1 lesions" ([39], p.745) must be vulnerable to critique. Attempts to model TGA pathogenesis should rightly be predicated on hippocampal anatomy but need to take account of more than simply CA1 (Sect. 9.7).

5.1.2.7   Other MR Findings

A study using high-resolution T2-reversed MR imaging in 15 patients who had recovered from TGA found hippocampal cavities in all patients, bilateral in eight, of frequency and size greater than in normal controls [59]. The rounded shape of these cavities was said to resemble the appearances seen in specimens of hypoxia-related hippocampal CA1 necrosis, prompting the view that the changes seen in TGA patients might represent neuronal loss within the hippocampal CA1 area, an observation which might have prognostic implications. However, Bartsch et al. [10] argued that these cavities were in the hippocampal sulcus, outside the CA1 region. Uttner et al. found no difference in cognitive performance in TGA patients with and without hippocampal cavities or in comparison to healthy controls (tested a median of >3 years post-TGA), although they confirmed the increased incidence of hippo-campal cavities in TGA patients [60], as did Park et al. [33].

Functional MR imaging has also been used to assess patients with TGA (Sect. 5.2.6).

5.1.3   Voxel-Based Morphometry (VBM) and Diffusion Tensor Imaging (DTI)

Advanced structural imaging techniques such as voxel-based morphometry (VBM) and diffusion tensor imaging (DTI) are research tools which permit assessment of indices such as cortical thickness and structural connectivity. DTI can be used to assess white matter microstructure in terms of its fractional anisotropy and mean diffusivity.

VBM showed significant differences in limbic structures including the hippo-campus between patients with TGA and controls, changes which were thought possibly to contribute to the vulnerability of memory pathways [33].

Using DTI, Moon et al. initially reported evidence suggesting disrupted neuronal integrity of cingulum bundle fibres in TGA [61] but subsequently reported no disruptions in the structural connectivity of the memory pathway in patients with recurrent TGA, suggesting no effect of recurrent events on brain microstructure [62].

Park et al. undertook DTI in recovered TGA patients and found no global differences with healthy controls and no differences in fractional anisotropy and mean diffusivity but did find reorganisation of network hubs [63]. These findings suggested the possibility that developmentally defined alterations in brain networks might predispose to TGA. Hodel et al. used DTI to show decreased structural connectivity in the limbic system in TGA patients with associated lower cortical thickness, at both acute (mean 44 h post-onset) and recovery (mean 35 days) stages [64]. Regional changes in cortical thickness and cortical volumes in TGA patients were also reported by Kim et al. [65]

Wang et al. found reduced fractional anisotropy in the hippocampus 3 months after recovery from TGA, but not at 2 weeks, suggesting the possibility of microstructural changes in hippocampus [66].

Lee et al. performed volumetric analysis and structural covariance network analysis in TGA patients and found no significant differences with healthy controls in global structural covariance network. However, the subgroup of patients with recurrent TGA did show significant alterations in this network, as well as in an intrahippocampal circuit which was also affected in single episode TGA patients. The authors suggested that these changes in connectivity could be relevant to TGA pathogenesis [67]. The same group of investigators also reported significant differences in functional networks in several brain regions according to TGA recurrence [68].

5.2 Functional Neuroimaging

5.2.1 Single-Photon Emission Computed Tomography (SPECT)

Of the various functional imaging modalities, single-photon emission computed tomography using 99mTechnetium hexamethylpropylene amine oxime (99mTc HMPAO-SPECT) to assess cerebral perfusion has generally been the most widely available resource and hence the most likely to be deployed in cases of TGA. The low spatial resolution of SPECT imaging compares unfavourably to MR imaging.

SPECT studies have generally shown decreased perfusion, in temporal lobe(s), frontal regions and parietotemporal regions, during attacks of TGA, with recovered perfusion seen in delayed imaging (e.g. [69–78]).

However, reports have also appeared of thalamic hypoperfusion [74, 75, 79–81] and global cerebral hypoperfusion [82]. Other reports have presented findings of hyperperfusion, of medial temporal lobe [83] and right parahippocampal gyrus ([84], case 1).

Lampl et al. found that SPECT remained abnormal at 3 and 12 months in three patients with recurrent TGA, whereas perfusion abnormalities resolved in patients with a first episode of TGA [73], observations which may be relevant to the prognosis of TGA (Sect. 6.2).

SPECT with 99mTc-ethyl cysteinate dimer (ECD) has also shown significant hypoperfusion acutely in left hippocampus, left thalamus and bilateral cerebellum, with restoration of perfusion in follow-up scans [85].

Examining MR and SPECT imaging in a series of TGA patients, Park et al. found that those with more anterior MR-DWI changes (especially hippocampal head) had associated SPECT hypoperfusion in the anterior frontal and temporal areas, whereas those with posterior MR-DWI changes (especially hippocampal tail) were associated with SPECT hypoperfusion in the posterior temporal, parietal, occipital and cerebellar areas, consistent with two parallel pathways between hippocampus and neocortex [86]. This observation, if corroborated, might explain some of the heterogeneity previously observed in SPECT imaging in TGA.

SPECT imaging in TGA has been superseded by MR imaging for a number of reasons: the low resolution and non-diagnostic nature of SPECT images and the now near ubiquity of access to acute MR imaging.

5.2.2 Positron Emission Tomography (PET)

Positron emission tomography (PET) may be used to assess cerebral blood flow and metabolism. The earliest PET studies in TGA were those of Oghino et al. [87] and Fujii et al. [88], undertaken several days to weeks after the attack.

A case study of a patient in the "acute (early recovery)" phase of TGA found a matched reduction in cerebral blood flow and oxygen consumption over the entire right lateral frontal cortex with an associated, less significant, reduction in ipsilateral thalamic and lentiform nucleus metabolism, but with sparing of the hippocampal area. Changes had resolved by the time of a follow-up scan 3 months later [89]. Further PET studies from this research group included a 59-year-old woman whose imaging showed reduced cerebral metabolic rate for oxygen and oxygen extraction fraction over the left cortical convexity, with metabolic rate particularly reduced in the left frontal and temporal regions, as well as over the left lenticular nucleus, but the hippocampal area appeared unremarkable. Findings were thought to indicate flow-metabolism uncoupling [90]. Two further patients examined with PET during TGA attacks showed significant changes in the amygdala (right or left) and left posterior hippocampus [91]. The findings suggested vascular disturbance during TGA attacks. Gonzalez-Martinez et al. reported left hippocampal hypometabolism following a tracer injection 2 h after onset of TGA [92].

PET studies conducted after TGA episodes have suggested better preservation of cerebral blood flow and oxygen metabolism compared with TIA patients [88]. Jia et al. reported "low metabolism in local areas related to memory in 2 of 3 patients" examined with PET at "different periods during recovery" [93].

5.2.3 CT Perfusion (CTP) Imaging

CT perfusion (CTP) imaging may be used for the early diagnosis of acute ischaemic stroke and TIA. In a single-centre study of CTP in 30 TGA patients, all had normal findings with respect to the hippocampi [94].

5.2.4   MR Spectroscopy (MRS)

Proton MR spectroscopy (1H-MRS) is a form of functional imaging which permits analysis of metabolites such as creatine (Cr), lactate, N-acetyl aspartate (NAA; a neuronal marker) and myoinositol (a marker of glial cells). One single patient study showed no changes in these markers [95]. However, Bartsch et al. performed focal MR spectroscopy of hippocampal CA1 lesions. In 4 of 7 TGA patients studied, the typical MR-DWI changes in the CA1 sector of the hippocampus were seen. MRS of diffusion lesions showed a lactate peak, a marker of anaerobic glycolysis, in three of four patients, but not in patients without a diffusion lesion. The NAA/Cr ratio was normal, suggesting no neuronal loss. The changes were thought to indicate acute metabolic stress of CA1 neurones [57].

5.2.5   Perfusion-Weighted MR Imaging

Perfusion-weighted MR imaging (dynamic susceptibility contrast perfusion-weighted MRI) may be used to assess cerebral perfusion in TGA, although this has more usually been assessed using SPECT and PET imaging (Sect. 5.2.1 and 5.2.2 respectively). No perfusion alterations were observed by visual inspection of perfusion-weighted MR imaging in five TGA patients, but group differences were found versus controls, with lower blood flow values bilaterally in the hippocampus, in the left thalamus and globus pallidus, as well as bilaterally in the putamen and the left caudate nucleus [96].

Shimizu et al. investigated TGA patients with conventional MR imaging as well as neurite orientation dispersion and density imaging (NODDI) and arterial spin labelling (ASL). They found no obvious microstructural or perfusion abnormalities in the hippocampus in DWI+ TGA patients, suggesting that neither destructive damage nor perfusion abnormalities were related to diffusion-restricted lesions [97]. Kim et al. found no differences in cerebral blood flow between single episode and recurrent TGA using MR-ASL [98].

5.2.6   Functional MRI (fMRI)

LaBar et al. used functional MRI (fMRI) to assess the integrity of temporal lobe activity during and after an episode of TGA using a visual scene encoding task. The findings were of deficits in a temporo-limbic circuit which recovered with time. During the amnesic state, the precentral gyrus and posterior parietal cortex were utilised more than after recovery from TGA. The authors suggested that frontoparietal areas recruited during the amnesic state may indicate a compensatory strategy using visuospatial or working memory capabilities. A reduction in responses in extrastriate cortex with repeated testing suggested the possibility of intact visual priming in TGA [99].

A similar fMRI study reported by Westmacott et al. showed no medial temporal activation associated with encoding of new scenes or recognition of old scenes during the amnesic period. However, there was strong hippocampal activation during attempted recognition despite unsuccessful retrieval. These changes had normalised at 3-month follow-up [100].

Peer et al. used resting-state fMRI in the acute phase of TGA in 12 patients to demonstrate a significant reduction in the functional connectivity of the episodic memory network, not just the hippocampus, which was reversible on recovery [101].

Zidda et al. showed reduced functional connectivity in executive network and hippocampus using fMRI in acute TGA compared to controls and recovered TGA patients, the latter two groups showing no significant differences [102].

Kim et al. [68] reported transiently greater functional connectivity in the salience network in TGA patients undergoing resting-state fMRI and lower functional connectivity in the default mode network, with preserved connectivity in the central executive network. The changes normalised by 3 months post-event.

5.3   Summary and Recommendations

Since TGA is a clinical diagnosis, no specific neuroimaging investigations are indicated. However, if there is diagnostic uncertainty, then investigations may be required to explore and refine the differential diagnosis. Neuroimaging may be required if there is a clinical suspicion of stroke. Of these investigations, diffusion-weighted magnetic resonance imaging is currently the most helpful. Focal punctate areas of signal change may be seen in the hippocampus, most often in the CA1 region, with the detection rate increasing between 1 and 4 days post-TGA and when using thin slice imaging. Whether or not these imaging changes leave long-term sequelae that might impact the prognosis of TGA, examined in the next chapter, remains uncertain, although some intriguing evidence to suggest altered network connectivity in recurrent TGA has emerged.

References

1. Riddoch D, Drolc Z. The value of brain scanning. Postgrad Med J. 1972;48:231–5.
2. Hodges JR, Warlow CP. Syndromes of transient amnesia: towards a classification. A study of 153 cases. J Neurol Neurosurg Psychiatry. 1990;53:834–43.
3. Caplan LB. [sic]. Transient global amnesia. In: Frederiks JAM, editor. Handbook of clinical neurology. Volume 1 (45). Clinical neuropsychology. Amsterdam: Elsevier Science Publishers; 1985. p. 205–18.
4. Hodges JR. Transient amnesia. Clinical and neuropsychological aspects. London: WB Saunders; 1991.

5. Morris Z, Whiteley WN, Longstreth WT, et al. Incidental findings on brain magnetic resonance imaging: systematic review and meta-analysis. BMJ. 2009;339:547–50.
6. Gass A, Gaa J, Hirsch J, Schwartz A, Hennerici MG. Lack of evidence of acute ischemic tissue change in transient global amnesia on single-shot echo-planar diffusion-weighted MRI. Stroke. 1999;30:2070–2.
7. Huber R, Aschoff AJ, Ludolph AC, Riepe MW. Transient global amnesia. Evidence against vascular ischemic etiology from diffusion weighted imaging. J Neurol. 2002;249:1520–4.
8. Alberici E, Pichiecchio A, Caverzasi E, et al. Transient global amnesia: hippocampal magnetic resonance imaging abnormalities. Funct Neurol. 2008;23:149–52.
9. Ay H, Furie KL, Yamada K, Koroshetz WJ. Diffusion-weighted MRI characterizes the ischemic lesion in transient global amnesia. Neurology. 1998;51:901–3.
10. Bartsch T, Alfke K, Stingele R, et al. Selective affection of hippocampal CA-1 neurons in patients with transient global amnesia without long-term sequelae. Brain. 2006;129:2874–84.
11. Bartsch T, Alfke K, Deuschl G, Jansen O. Evolution of hippocampal CA-1 diffusion lesions in transient global amnesia. Ann Neurol. 2007;62:475–80.
12. Bartsch T, Schonfeld R, Muller FJ, et al. Focal lesions of human hippocampal CA1 neurons in transient global amnesia impair place memory. Science. 2010;328:1412–5.
13. Cianfoni A, Tartaglione T, Gaudino S, et al. Hippocampal magnetic resonance imaging abnormalities in transient global amnesia. Arch Neurol. 2005;62:1468–9.
14. Enzinger C, Thimary F, Kapeller P, et al. Transient global amnesia: diffusion-weighted imaging lesions and cerebrovascular disease. Stroke. 2008;39:2219–25.
15. Felix MM, Castro LH, Maia AC Jr, da Rocha AJ. Evidence of acute ischaemic tissue change in transient global amnesia in magnetic resonance imaging: case report and literature review. J Neuroimaging. 2005;15:203–5.
16. Fernandez A, Rincon F, Mazer SP, Elkind MS. Magnetic resonance imaging changes in a patient with migraine attack and transient global amnesia after cardiac catheterization. CNS Spectr. 2005;10:980–3.
17. Inamura T, Nakazaki K, Yasuda O, et al. A lesion diagnosed by MRI in a case of transient global amnesia [in Japanese]. No To Shinkei. 2002;54:419–22.
18. Matsui M, Imamura T, Sakamoto S, Ishii K, Kazui H, Mori E. Transient global amnesia: increased signal intensity in the right hippocampus on diffusion-weighted magnetic resonance imaging. Neuroradiology. 2002;44:235–8.
19. Sedlaczek O, Hirsch JG, Grips E, et al. Detection of delayed focal MR changes in the lateral hippocampus in transient global amnesia. Neurology. 2004;62:2165–70.
20. Strupp M, Brüning R, Wu RH, Deimling M, Reiser M, Brandt T. Diffusion-weighted MRI in transient global amnesia: elevated signal intensity in the left mesial temporal lobe in 7 out of 10 patients. Ann Neurol. 1998;43:164–70.
21. Weon YC, Kim JH, Lee JS, Kim SY. Optimal diffusion-weighted imaging protocol for lesion detection in transient global amnesia. AJNR Am J Neuroradiol. 2008;29:1324–8.
22. Wilkinson T, Geranmayeh F, Dassan P, Janssen JC. Neuroimaging in transient global amnesia. Pract Neurol. 2013;13:56–7.
23. Winbeck K, Etgen T, von Einsiedel HG, Röttinger M, Sander D. DWI in transient global amnesia and TIA: proposal for an ischaemic origin of TGA. J Neurol Neurosurg Psychiatry. 2005;76:438–41.
24. Woolfenden AR, O'Brien MW, Schwartzberg RE, Norbash AM, Tong DC. Diffusion-weighted MRI in transient global amnesia precipitated by cerebral angiography. Stroke. 1997;28:2311–4.
25. Ahn S, Kim W, Lee YS, et al. Transient global amnesia: seven years of experience with diffusion-weighted imaging in an emergency department. Eur Neurol. 2011;65:123–8.
26. Higashida K, Okazaki S, Todo K, et al. A multicenter study of transient global amnesia for the better detection of magnetic resonance imaging abnormalities. Eur J Neurol. 2020;27:2117–24.

27. Kim J, Kwon Y, Yang Y, et al. Clinical experience of modified diffusion-weighted imaging protocol for lesion detection in transient global amnesia: an 8-year large-scale clinical study. J Neuroimaging. 2014;24:331–7.
28. Ryoo I, Kim JH, Kim S, Choi BS, Jung C, Hwang SI. Lesion detectability on diffusion-weighted imaging in transient global amnesia: the influence of imaging timing and magnetic field strength. Neuroradiology. 2012;54:329–34.
29. Scheel M, Malkowsky C, Klingebiel R, Schreiber SJ, Bohner G. Magnetic resonance imaging in transient global amnesia: lessons learned from 198 cases. Clin Neuroradiol. 2012;22:335–40.
30. Szabo K, Hoyer C, Caplan LR, et al. Diffusion-weighted MRI in transient global amnesia and its diagnostic implications. Neurology. 2020;95:e206–12.
31. Lim SJ, Kim M, Suh CH, Kim SY, Shim WH, Kim SJ. Diagnostic yield of diffusion-weighted brain magnetic resonance imaging in patients with transient global amnesia: a systematic review and meta-analysis. Korean J Radiol. 2021;22:1680–9.
32. Wong ML, Silva LO, Gerberi DJ, Edlow JA, Dubosh NM. Sensitivity of diffusion-weighted magnetic resonance imaging in transient global amnesia as a function of time from onset. Acad Emerg Med. 2021; https://doi.org/10.1111/acem.14390. Online ahead of print
33. Park KM, Han YH, Kim TH, et al. Pre-existing structural abnormalities of the limbic system in transient global amnesia. J Clin Neurosci. 2015;22:843–7.
34. Auyeung M, Tsoi TH, Cheung CM, et al. Association of diffusion weighted imaging abnormalities and recurrence in transient global amnesia. J Clin Neurosci. 2011;18:531–4.
35. Lorente de Nó R. Studies on the structure of the cerebral cortex. II. Continuation of the study of the ammonic system. J Psychol Neurol. 1934;46:113–77.
36. Lee HY, Kim JH, Weon YC, et al. Diffusion-weighted imaging in transient global amnesia exposes the CA1 region of the hippocampus. Neuroradiology. 2007;49:481–7.
37. Döhring J, Schmuck A, Bartsch T. Stress-related factors in the emergence of transient global amnesia with hippocampal lesions. Front Behav Neurosci. 2014;8:287.
38. Yang Y, Kim S, Kim JH. Ischemic evidence of transient global amnesia: location of the lesion in the hippocampus. J Clin Neurol. 2008;4:59–66.
39. Hanert A, Pedersen A, Bartsch T. Transient hippocampal CA1 lesions in humans impair pattern separation performance. Hippocampus. 2019;29:736–47.
40. Tarazona LR, Martinez EL, Llopis CM. Transient global amnesia with extra-hippocampal lesion and a normal cardiovascular study. Can J Neurol Sci. 2021;24:1–2. https://doi.org/10.1017/cjn.2021.116. Online ahead of print
41. Morena J, Kamdar HA, Adeli A. Cerebellar ischemia presenting as transient global amnesia. Cogn Behav Neurol. 2021;34:319–22.
42. Ganeshan R, Betz M, Scheitz JF, et al. Frequency of silent brain infarction in transient global amnesia. J Neurol. 2022;269:1422–6.
43. Piffer S, Nannoni S, Maulucci F et al. The transient global amnesia-hippocampal punctate diffusion lesion spectrum: atypical clinical and radiological presentations. A case series and systematic review. 2021; submitted.
44. Ueno H, Naka H, Ohshita T, Wakabayashi S, Matsumoto M. Serial changes in delayed focal hippocampal lesions in patients with transient global amnesia. Hiroshima J Med Sci. 2010;59:77–81.
45. Paech D, Kuder TA, Roßmanith C, et al. What remains after transient global amnesia (TGA)? An ultra-high field 7T magnetic resonance imaging study of the hippocampus. Eur J Neurol. 2020;27:406–9.
46. Lee SY, Kim WJ, Suh SH, Oh SH, Lee KY. Higher lesion detection by 3.0T MRI in patient with transient global amnesia. Yonsei Med J. 2009;50:211–4.
47. Choi BS, Kim JH, Jung C, Kim SY. High-resolution diffusion-weighted imaging increases lesion detectability in patients with transient global amnesia. AJNR Am J Neuroradiol. 2012;33:1771–4.

48. Larner AJ. The 2x2 matrix. Contingency, confusion and the metrics of binary classification. London: Springer; 2021.
49. Bartsch T, Döhring J, Reuter S, et al. Selective neuronal vulnerability of human hippocampal CA1 neurons: lesion evolution, temporal course, and pattern of hippocampal damage in diffusion-weighted MR imaging. J Cereb Blood Flow Metab. 2015;35:1836–45.
50. Förster A, Al-Zghloul M, Wenz H, Böhme J, Groden C, Neumaier-Probst E. Isolated punctuate hippocampal infarction and transient global amnesia are indistinguishable by means of MRI. Int J Stroke. 2017;12:292–6.
51. Park JH, Oh CG, Kim SH, Lee S, Jang J. Hippocampal lesions of diffusion weighted magnetic resonance image in patients with headache without symptoms of transient global amnesia. Dement Neurocogn Disord. 2017;16:87–90.
52. Jeong M, Jin J, Kim JH, Moon Y, Choi JW, Kim HY. Incidental hippocampal hyperintensity on diffusion-weighted MRI: individual susceptibility to transient global amnesia. Neurologist. 2017;22:103–6.
53. Larner AJ. Diagnostic test accuracy studies in dementia. A pragmatic approach. 2nd ed. London: Springer; 2019.
54. Bartsch T, Döhring J, Rohr A, Jansen O, Deuschl G. CA1 neurons in the human hippocampus are critical for autobiographical memory, mental time travel, and autonoetic consciousness. Proc Natl Acad Sci U S A. 2011;108:17562–7.
55. Kartsounis LD, Rudge P, Stevens JM. Bilateral lesions of CA1 and CA2 fields of the hippocampus are sufficient to cause a severe amnesic syndrome in humans. J Neurol Neurosurg Psychiatry. 1995;59:95–8.
56. Zola-Morgan S, Squire LR, Amaral DG. Human amnesia and the medial temporal region: enduring memory impairment following a bilateral lesion limited to field CA1 of the hippocampus. J Neurosci. 1986;6:2950–67.
57. Bartsch T, Alfke K, Wolff S, Rohr A, Jansen O, Deuschl G. Focal MR spectroscopy of hippocampal CA-1 lesions in transient global amnesia. Neurology. 2008;70:1030–5.
58. Carpenter RHS. Neurophysiology. 3rd ed. London: Arnold; 1996.
59. Nakada T, Kwee IL, Fujii Y, Knight RT. High-field, T2 reversed MRI of the hippocampus in transient global amnesia. Neurology. 2005;64:1170–4.
60. Uttner I, Weber S, Freund W, et al. Hippocampal cavities are not associated with cognitive impairment in transient global amnesia. Eur J Neurol. 2011;18:882–7.
61. Moon Y, Oh J, Kwon KJ, Han SH. Transient global amnesia: only in already disrupted neuronal integrity of memory network? J Neurol Sci. 2016;368:187–90.
62. Moon Y, Moon WJ, Han SH. The structural connectivity of the recurrent transient global amnesia. Acta Neurol Scand. 2016;134:160–4.
63. Park KM, Lee BI, Kim SE. Is transient global amnesia a network disease? Eur Neurol. 2018;80:345–54.
64. Hodel J, Leclerc X, Zuber M, et al. Structural connectivity and cortical thickness alterations in transient global amnesia. AJNR Am J Neuroradiol. 2020;41:798–803.
65. Kim HC, Lee BI, Kim SE, Park KM. Cortical morphology in patients with transient global amnesia. Brain Behav. 2017;7:e00872.
66. Wang X, Zhang R, Wei W, et al. Long-term sequelae of hippocampal lesions in patients with transient global amnesia: a multiparametric MRI study. J Magn Reson Imaging. 2018;47:1350–8.
67. Lee DA, Lee S, Kim DW, Lee H, Park KM. Effective connectivity alteration according to recurrence in transient global amnesia. Neuroradiology. 2021;63:1441–9.
68. Kim GH, Kim BR, Chun MY, Park KD, Lim SM, Jeong JH. Aberrantly higher functional connectivity in the salience network is associated with transient global amnesia. Sci Rep. 2021;11:20598.
69. Bucuk M, Muzur A, Willheim K, Jurjevic A, Tomic Z, Tuskan ML. Make love to forget: two cases of transient global amnesia triggered by sexual intercourse. Coll Anthropol. 2004;28:899–905.

70. Evans J, Wilson B, Wraight EP, Hodges JR. Neuropsychological and SPECT scan findings during and after transient global amnesia: evidence for the differential impairment of remote episodic memory. J Neurol Neurosurg Psychiatry. 1993;56:1227–30.

71. Jovin TG, Vitti RA, McCluskey LF. Evolution of temporal lobe hypoperfusion in transient global amnesia: a serial single photon emission computed tomography study. J Neuroimaging. 2000;10:238–41.

72. Laloux P, Brichant C, Cauwe F, Decoster P. Technetium-99m HM-PAO single photon emission computed tomography imaging in transient global amnesia. Arch Neurol. 1992;49:543–6.

73. Lampl Y, Sadeh M, Lorberboym M. Transient global amnesia—not always a benign process. Acta Neurol Scand. 2004;110:75–9.

74. Sakashita Y, Sugimoto T, Taki S, Matsuda H. Abnormal cerebral blood flow following transient global amnesia. J Neurol Neurosurg Psychiatry. 1993;56:1327.

75. Schmidtke K, Reinhardt M, Krause T. Cerebral hypoperfusion during transient global amnesia: findings with HMPAO SPECT. J Nucl Med. 1998;39:155–9.

76. Stillhard G, Landis T, Schiess R, Regard M, Sialer G. Bitemporal hypoperfusion in transient global amnesia: 99m-Tc-HM-PAO SPECT and neuropsychological findings during and after an attack. J Neurol Neurosurg Psychiatry. 1990;53:339–42.

77. Tanabe H, Hashikawa K, Nakagawa Y, et al. Memory loss due to transient hypoperfusion in the medial temporal lobes including hippocampus. Acta Neurol Scand. 1991;84:22–7. [Erratum Acta Neurol Scand. 1991;84:463]

78. Warren JD, Chatterton B, Thompson PD. A SPECT study of the anatomy of transient global amnesia. J Clin Neurosci. 2000;7:57–9.

79. Goldenberg G. Transient global amnesia. In: Baddeley AD, Wilson BA, Watts FN, editors. Handbook of memory disorders. Chichester: John Wiley; 1995. p. 113–4.

80. Goldenberg G, Podreka I, Pfaffelmeyer N, Wessely P, Deecke L. Thalamic ischemia in transient global amnesia: a SPECT study. Neurology. 1991;41:1748–52.

81. Nardone R, Buffone EC, Matullo MF, Tezzon F. Motor cortex excitability in transient global amnesia. J Neurol. 2004;251:42–6.

82. Yamane Y, Ishii K, Shimizu K, et al. Global cerebral hypoperfusion in a patient with transient global amnesia. J Comput Assist Tomogr. 2008;32:415–7.

83. Matsuda H, Higashi S, Tsuji S, et al. High resolution Tc-99m HMPAO SPECT in a patient with transient global amnesia. Clin Nucl Med. 1993;18:46–9.

84. Asada T, Matsuda H, Morooka T, Nakano S, Kimura M, Uno M. Quantitative single photon emission tomography analysis for the diagnosis of transient global amnesia: adaptation of statistical parametric mapping. Psychiatry Clin Neurosci. 2000;54:691–4.

85. Kim BS, Cho SS, Choi JY, Kim YH. Transient global amnesia: a study with Tc-99m ECD SPECT shortly after symptom onset and recovery. Diagn Interv Radiol. 2016;22:476–80.

86. Park YH, Jang JW, Yang Y, Kim JE, Kim S. Reflections of two parallel pathways between the hippocampus and neocortex in transient global amnesia: a cross-sectional study using DWI and SPECT. PLoS One. 2013;8:e67447.

87. Oghino Y, Yokoi F, Nishio T, Sunohara N, Satayoshi E. Positron emission tomography in two cases of transient global amnesia [in Japanese]. Rinsho Shinkeigaku. 1989;29:599–605.

88. Fujii K, Sadoshima S, Ishitsuka T, et al. Regional cerebral blood flow and metabolism in patients with transient global amnesia: a positron emission tomography study. J Neurol Neurosurg Psychiatry. 1989;52:622–30.

89. Baron JC, Petit-Taboué MC, Le Doze F, Desgranges B, Ravenel N, Marchal G. Right frontal cortex hypometabolism in transient global amnesia. A PET study. Brain. 1994;117:545–52.

90. Eustache F, Desgranges B, Petit-Taboué MC, et al. Transient global amnesia: implicit/explicit memory dissociation and PET assessment of brain perfusion and oxygen metabolism in the acute stage. J Neurol Neurosurg Psychiatry. 1997;63:357–67.

91. Guillery B, Desgranges B, de la Sayette V, Landeau B, Eustache F, Baron JC. Transient global amnesia: concomitant episodic memory and positron emission tomography assessment in two additional patients. Neurosci Lett. 2002;325:62–6.

92. Gonzalez-Martinez V, Comte F, de Verbizier D, Carlander B. Transient global amnesia: con-
     cordant hippocampal abnormalities on positron emission tomography and magnetic reso-
     nance imaging. Arch Neurol. 2010;67:510–1.
 93. Jia J, Wang L, Yin L, Tang H. Contrast study on cognitive function with MRI and positron
     emission tomography imaging in transient global amnesia. Chin Med J. 2002;115:1321–3.
 94. Meyer IA, Wintermark M, Démonet JF, Michel P. CTP in transient global amnesia: a single-
     center experience of 30 patients. AJNR Am J Neuroradiol. 2015;36:1830–3.
 95. Zorzon M, Longo R, Mase G, Biasutti E, Vitrani B, Cazzato G. Proton magnetic resonance
     spectroscopy during transient global amnesia. J Neurol Sci. 1998;156:78–82.
 96. Förster A, Al-Zghloul M, Kerl HU, Böhme J, Mürle B, Groden C. Value of dynamic suscep-
     tibility contrast perfusion MRI in the acute phase of transient global amnesia. PLoS One.
     2015;10(3):e0122537.
 97. Shimizu K, Hara S, Hori M, et al. Transient global amnesia: a diffusion and perfusion MRI
     study. J Neuroimaging. 2020;30:828–32.
 98. Kim J, Lee DA, Kim HC, Lee H, Park KM. Brain networks in patients with isolated or recur-
     rent transient global amnesia. Acta Neurol Scand. 2021;144:465–72.
 99. LaBar KS, Gitelman DR, Parrish TB, Mesulam M-M. Functional changes in temporal lobe
     activity during transient global amnesia. Neurology. 2002;58:638–41.
100. Westmacott R, Silver FL, McAndrews MP. Understanding medial temporal activation in
     memory tasks: evidence from fMRI of encoding and recognition in a case of transient global
     amnesia. Hippocampus. 2008;18:317–25.
101. Peer M, Nitzan M, Goldberg I, et al. Reversible functional connectivity disturbances during
     transient global amnesia. Ann Neurol. 2014;75:634–43.
102. Zidda F, Griebe M, Ebert A, et al. Resting-state connectivity alterations during transient
     global amnesia. Neuroimage Clin. 2019;23:101869.

Chapter 6
Prognosis and Management of TGA

Abstract This chapter considers the prognosis and management of TGA. Generally, prognosis is benign, although some mild deficits of memory function may persist as well as a gap for the period of TGA. There is a finite recurrence rate, around 3–6% per year, and it may possibly be the case that recurrent TGA is not as benign as single-episode TGA. Uncertainties remain about long-term risks of developing dementia, epilepsy, stroke and depression.

Keywords Cognition · Recurrent TGA · Epilepsy

A number of studies investigating the prognosis of TGA have appeared (e.g. [1–13].), with variable methods of case ascertainment and duration of follow-up. Generally, these have confirmed the benign outlook in TGA, as has a systematic review [14] although subtle cognitive deficits may persist and there may possibly be increased risk of dementia and epilepsy.

6.1 Recovery and Persisting Cognitive Deficit

In most patients with TGA, recovery of memory function is rapid, with apparent restoration to normal with the exception of the amnesic episode per se (see Sect. 1.1, Sect. 2.1.5 and Sect. 4.1.3). However, some formal studies have suggested that memory function may not return entirely to normal.

In the recovery phase of an acute attack of TGA (post-acute phase), retrograde amnesia recovers before anterograde amnesia, but the shrinkage of the former may be heterogeneous, with or without a temporal gradient [15]. Kapur et al. attempted to fractionate memory tests in patients recovering from TGA and found that resolution of a naming deficit more closely paralleled recovery from retrograde amnesia rather than anterograde amnesia. Within retrograde amnesia for public events, there was a temporal gradient of memory loss, with more recent events affected to a greater degree than earlier events. Within anterograde amnesia, picture recognition memory preceded recovery of story recall memory [16].

Persistent retrograde memory deficit after TGA has been described on occasion. Roman-Campos et al. presented a patient with a 5- to 10-year period of retrograde amnesia after the acute episode. However, these authors reported EEG changes suggestive of a left temporal lobe lesion [17], and hence, the possibility that this was an epileptic amnesic attack, rather than TGA, cannot be excluded. Mazzucchi et al. reported deficits in verbal long-term memory and verbal IQ in sixteen TGA patients [18], and Cattaino et al. reported permanent memory impairment in 15/30 patients followed up for a mean interval of 20 months [19]. However, the majority of patients in this study had vascular risk factors, prompting concern that some of these patients suffered from amnesic stroke rather than TGA ([20], p.37–8). A review by Mueller dating from 1989 included eight studies in the literature encompassing 622 TGA patients and 122 patients from a personal survey and reached the conclusion that a "residual syndrome of disturbed long term verbal memory may be seen even after a single attack" [8].

Hodges and Oxbury ([21]; see also [22], p.90–6) studied 41 TGA patients 6 months after their attacks. Compared to age-, sex- and IQ-matched controls, there was no evidence of general intellectual decline, and immediate (working) memory for both verbal and non-verbal material was normal, but there was inferior performance on long-term memory tests (paragraph recall). Remote memory was also impaired, as assessed by the Famous Faces test (identifying famous people from previous decades) and famous events (dating significant previous events; recognition, an easier test, was not impaired). The temporal gradient observed in dating famous events seen in the acute phase (Sect. 4.1.1.3) was not seen in the 6-month follow-up. On the Crovitz test of cued autobiographical memory, there were impairments. Longer-term non-verbal memory, assessed by recall of the Rey–Osterrieth Complex Figure and by learning a supraspan block tapping sequence, was intact. Hence, the anterograde memory deficit appeared to be material-specific. The authors posited a mild hippocampal–diencephalic dysfunction preferentially affecting left-sided structures.

Le Pira et al. documented cognitive dysfunction after clinical recovery in a group of 14 TGA patients compared to matched controls. Quantitative differences were found in performance on the California Verbal Learning Test (CVLT) and the Rey–Osterrieth Complex Figure Test, with reduced categorical learning and attention that were ascribed to a prefrontal impairment [23].

Guillery-Girard et al. investigated 32 patients 13–67 months post-TGA attack and reported deficits in the retrieval of recent semantic information and episodic memories which they thought most likely to be due to difficulty accessing memories [24].

Testing patients at a mean of 3 years post-TGA, Uttner et al. found no differences in neuropsychological assessment between TGA patients and controls [12]. In a subsequent study, no differences were found in patients with or without acute MR-DWI changes versus healthy controls 2 years after TGA [13].

Jäger et al. administered a recognition memory task for faces and words to eleven TGA patients during the post-acute phase and to eleven matched controls. They sought to examine dual-process models of recognition memory, which posit that recollection and familiarity are mediated by hippocampal and extra-hippocampal brain regions, respectively, hypothesising that because of the changes seen in the hippocampus on diffusion-weighted magnetic resonance imaging (MR-DWI) in TGA patients (Sect. 5.1.2), the former may be more impaired than the latter. They found impaired recollection in the TGA patients' memory for words, but no difference between TGA patients and controls in familiarity-based recognition memory, suggesting that TGA has selective effects on specific recognition memory subprocesses, consistent with a dual-process model [25].

Noël et al. studied 19 patients one year after TGA and found that mild anterograde memory deficits could be detected. As might be anticipated, patients with evidence for depression or anxiety (see Sect. 6.3.5) did worse. Although the mild post-TGA episodic memory disorder may be a consequence of TGA, the authors suggested that patients' emotional state might slow recovery processes [26].

Schöberl et al. used sophisticated tests of hippocampal function which indicated selective and prolonged deficits in allocentric (hippocampus-dependent) spatial navigation in patients following TGA, suggesting that damage had occurred within hippocampal circuits [27].

Fewer follow-up studies have been reported in possible variants of TGA (see Sect. 2.3 for descriptions of these phenotypes). Neuropsychological evaluation in transient topographical amnesia (TTA; Sect. 2.3.1) 6–12 months after recovery showed normal performance in all tasks but lower performance compared to controls in a test of spatial (geographical) orientation, but it was not known whether this deficit predated the TTA events [28]. One patient in the series of patients with TTA reported by Naranjo-Fernandez et al. [29] developed dementia six years after the acute episode.

In view of the mild impairment in verbal memory following TGA reported in some studies, the possibility that these patients may be at risk for long-term cognitive decline, manifesting as mild cognitive impairment or dementia, has been examined (Sect. 6.3.1).

6.2 Recurrence

In one of the earliest published reports of TGA, Morris Bender described isolated or single episodes of confusion with amnesia [30] and later emphasised the absence of recurrence [31]. However, the possibility of recurrence of TGA was mentioned in the early literature, for example by Guyotat and Courjon [32] and by Fisher and Adams [33]. However, it was the paper by Lou in 1968 which first made the possibility of recurrence of TGA explicit, although at least one patient in this series was almost certainly having ischaemic events [34].

Many subsequent reports of recurrent TGA have appeared (although not all can be accepted as such, especially those predating widespread application of Hodges and Warlow's 1990 diagnostic criteria [35]). Accounts include recurrence associated with sexual activity [36–38], at high altitude [39], as well as detail from the patient's perspective [40]. Recurrence has also been reported in transient topographical amnesia (TTA), a possible variant form of TGA (Sect. 2.3.1). Occurrence of up to three episodes was noted in 3/10 patients [41], with a mean number of episodes of 1.75, range 1–3 [29], although some patients are reported to have many episodes over many years [42].

6.2.1   Annual Recurrence Rate

Although numbers of studies have cited a "recurrence rate" for TGA, fewer have taken into account the duration and extent of patient follow-up and are thus able to calculate an annual recurrence rate (Table 6.1). These are for the most part prospective studies, and their findings suggest an annual TGA recurrence rate of around 3–6%. Mueller reviewed eight "representative" studies from the literature encompassing 622 TGA patients and 122 patients from a personal survey to produce a risk of recurrence of 3.4%/year [8].

Low recurrence rate is one factor which may assist in the differential diagnosis of TGA from transient epileptic amnesia (TEA) and from transient ischaemic attack (TIA) (see Table 3.3). Although occasional patients undoubtedly do suffer recurrent episodes of TGA (Case Study 2.1) [45], frequent recurrence of events labelled as TGA should certainly prompt careful diagnostic consideration, and possibly concern, for example the case reported by Rumpl and Rumpl [46], also associated with epileptic seizures, unilateral visual loss, hemiparesis and dysarthria (see also [47, 48]). Questions about the differential diagnosis, especially from epilepsy, may need to be reassessed (e.g. [49, 50]).

6.2.2   Recurrent TGA

Do patients with recurrent (definite or pure) TGA differ from those who experience only a single episode? A number of lines of evidence, both clinical and radiological, suggest this possibility, although the caveats concerning adequate differentiation from TEA must be borne in mind when assessing these accounts.

Table 6.1 Reports of annual recurrence rates of TGA

Reference	Study location	Annual recurrence rate
Hinge et al. (1986) [5]	Danish multicentre	4.7%
Hodges (1991) [22]	Oxford, UK	ca. 3%
Toledo et al. (2005) [43]	Barcelona, Spain	4.4%
Quinnette et al. (2006) [44]	Caen, France	5.8%

Gallassi et al. undertook neuropsychological tests in patients with single ($n = 31$) or multiple ($n = 10$) TGA episodes compared with matched controls ($n = 41$) and found that patients with multiple attacks showed more impairment in tasks addressing memory and visuoperceptual abilities than patients with single attacks who showed only immediate and long-term verbal memory impairments with respect to controls [51].

Lampl et al. found that acute brain hypoperfusion seen on SPECT imaging (Sect. 5.2.1) in 16 TGA patients returned to normal after 3 months in those patients experiencing a first episode of TGA, whereas perfusion remained abnormal at 3 and 12 months in three patients with recurrent TGA [52].

Toledo et al. compared "unique-TGA" cases ($n = 98$) with "recurrent-TGA" cases ($n = 26$) and found that the latter had the same vascular risk factors (Sect. 7.11) as a comparison group of TIA patients. Moreover, the recurrent-TGA patients had a significantly more frequent history of stroke and a trend to suffer new ischaemic events than patients in the unique-TGA group, prompting the authors to suggest that recurrent TGA should be considered a manifestation of ischaemic cerebrovascular disease [43]. However, in a later study these authors revised their view, finding no perfusion abnormalities, arterial stenoses or underlying cardioembolic disease in a series of 28 TGA patients [53].

Agosti et al. studied 85 TGA patients recruited over a 3-year period of whom 73 had a single episode and 12 (14.1%) had two episodes. A risk factor sum of recognised TGA triggers was calculated for each patient and this was higher for the recurrent group, who also had a higher frequency of carotid atheroma (41.8% vs. 15.1%, $p < 0.05$) and ischaemic heart disease (6.8% vs. 3.3%, $p < 0.02$) [54].

A magnetic resonance imaging study of TGA patients ($n = 27$) looking at diffusion-weighted abnormalities in the hippocampus (Sect. 5.1.2) found these in nine patients, with a higher association observed in patients with a second TGA attack compared to a first event. These authors concluded that patients with recurrent TGA had a significantly higher association of reversible MR-DWI abnormality [55].

Moon et al. undertook diffusion tensor imaging (Sect. 5.1.3) in seven patients with recurrent TGA and fourteen with single-episode TGA to examine the hypothesis that the former might have more disrupted structural connectivity and hence greater pre-existing vulnerability to TGA attacks. The study found no disruptions in the structural connectivity of the memory pathway in recurrent-TGA patients, suggesting that repeated hippocampal lesions associated with TGA do not affect the microstructure of the brain [56]. However, volumetric analyses (Sect. 5.1.3) have suggested the possibility of network alterations in connectivity in recurrent TGA [57, 58].

Summarising these disparate studies, there does appear to be some tentative, but not uniform, evidence that prognosis following recurrent TGA may differ from that following single-event or unique TGA, being less benign. Whether this subgroup can be recognised from the outset, i.e. after their first episode, on the basis of risk factor profiles or biomarkers, remains to be determined, but this might have implications for management.

6.2.3   Possible Risk Factors for Recurrent TGA

Are there specific risk factors for recurrence of TGA? Morris et al. examined over 1000 patients with TGA, of whom 13.7% had had at least one recurrence (maximum 9). They found a significant difference in age at first TGA episode between individuals with a single-episode (65.2 ± 10.0 years) compared to those with recurrent episodes (58.8 ± 10.3 years). In addition, a personal or family history of migraine was more prevalent in recurrent compared to isolated cases [59].

Alessandro et al. [60] reported that 8% of 203 TGA patients seen in Buenos Aires had a recurrence over a mean follow-up of 24 months. A personal history of migraine was more frequent in patients with than without recurrence.

Tynas and Panegyres followed up a cohort of 93 TGA cases of whom 16% had recurrence. Risk factors for recurrence were depression, previous head injury and a family history of dementia. Typical MR-DWI changes, observed in 24 patients, were not associated with outcomes in this patient cohort [61].

In a cohort of 70 TGA patients followed up for mean of 16.5 months, Oliveira et al. found TGA recurrence in 27%, and associated with female sex, depression, shorter duration of TGA episode and hippocampus hyperintensity on MR-DWI (although only 5 patients in the cohort had this change). Of these, a history of depression was the most important predictor [62].

Ganeshan et al. reported recurrence in 13/126 patients in their study, with no difference in percentage recurrence between those patients with and without additional non-hippocampal (silent) ischaemic lesions [63].

A systematic review by Liampas et al. found evidence for a relationship between recurrence risk and a personal or family history of migraine and a personal history of depression. Weaker evidence was found for a relationship with family history of dementia, personal history of head injury and MR-DWI hippocampal lesions. However, no relationship was found with EEG abnormalities, impaired jugular venous drainage, cardiovascular risk factors, atrial fibrillation or cardiovascular events [64].

6.2.4   Is Family History of TGA a Risk Factor
for Recurrent TGA?

A small number of patients reported in the TGA literature give a history of TGA episodes in other family members (Sect. 7.8). A patient reported from the author's clinic who had recurrent TGA and whose father reportedly also had recurrent TGA prompted the question as to whether or not a positive family history of TGA is a risk factor for recurrent-TGA episodes [65]. Following this publication, the author has received emails from other families with recurrent and familial TGA [66], which are summarised along with cases reported in the published literature in Table 6.2.

Table 6.2 Reports of familial cases of TGA with history of TGA recurrence (see Table 7.3 for reports of familial TGA cases)

Reference	TGA patient details	Recurrence history
Corston and Godwin-Austen (1982) [67]	Four male siblings, aged in 60s and 70s; three had TGA attacks in the context of exercise	2–3 attacks each
Munro and Loizou (1982) [68]	Two siblings (M:F) and their father, in 50s to 60s	2 attacks in index case (M), 3 in father
Dupuis et al. (1987) [69]	Twin sisters (probably monozygotic), attacks in 60s	2 attacks in first sister, aged 64 and 69, both attacks followed by severe migraine
Vyhnalek et al. (2008) [70]	Male, father and sister. Proband had migraine without aura from adolescence; no migraine in father or sister	Male had 2 episodes aged 52 and 54. Father and sister had single episodes
Segers-van Rijn and de Bruijn (2010) [71]	Four siblings (3F:1M) and possibly their mother, attacks after exercise (3) and air travel (1), and on birthday; attacks between 50s and 70s	One of the female siblings had history of two episodes
Maggioni et al. (2011) [72]	Two monozygotic twin brothers aged 50 and 49 at onset	Elder brother had 5-6 attacks per year during migraine without aura (MO) attacks; younger had four episodes all during MO
Larner 2017 [65]	Male; father also reportedly had TGA	Index case had two episodes, aged 61 and 64; father 2–3 episodes (uncertain)
Larner (2018) [66]	Two male siblings and their mother	Younger male sibling had three events, aged 60, 63, 66, first two after exercise (cycling)
Larner (2018) [66]	Two female siblings, both had history of migraine	Younger female sibling had two events, aged 54 and 55, second after sexual activity. Older sibling had single event, aged 60, after sexual activity
Larner (2019) (unpublished, personal communication)	Three siblings (1F:2M)	Female had 3 events aged 63, 68, 70, first after emotional upset, second after exercise. Single events in male siblings

In addition, Dupuis et al. [73] reported (in abstract) a higher recurrence rate (and history of migraine) in those TGA patients with a positive family history of TGA (21) compared to the whole cohort of 219 patients (24% vs 12.6%) seen over an extended period of time (1999–2016). Morris et al. reported a family history of TGA in 1.3% of their cohort with single-episode TGA and in 2.8% with recurrent TGA [59]. Liampas et al. found no relationship between TGA recurrence and family history of TGA [64]. However, given that both familial history and recurrence of TGA are likely to be underascertained, this possible link may merit further examination in prospective population-based studies.

6.3 Future Risk

Generally, TGA has been regarded as a benign event with respect to long-term prognosis. But in light of some of the aforementioned clinical and imaging findings (Sects. 6.1 and 6.2), it is pertinent to ask whether or not an episode or episodes of TGA may put patients at risk for future neurological problems. In other words, is the long-term prognosis of TGA entirely benign or not? This has been examined particularly for cognitive decline, stroke and epilepsy.

6.3.1 Cognitive Decline: Dementia and Mild Cognitive Impairment (MCI)

Because cognitive decline becomes increasingly prevalent with ageing, it is not surprising to encounter patients with cognitive impairment who have a prior history of an episode of TGA (especially so in view of the typical age at which TGA occurs; Sect. 7.4), without there necessarily being an implication that subsequence is consequence (see Case Studies 6.1 and 6.2), or in other words that dementia is "presenting" as TGA [74].

Case Study 6.1: Dementia Subsequent, but not Consequent, to TGA
A 73-year-old man was referred with a two-year history of progressive memory difficulties, corroborated by family members. On the Mini-Mental State Examination, he scored 22/30 and on the Addenbrooke's Cognitive Examination-Revised 60/100. MR brain imaging showed bilateral temporal lobe atrophy. A diagnosis of Alzheimer's disease was made. Nine years earlier, he had had an episode of memory loss after going for a swim one morning whilst on holiday, with resolution after about 7 h. He was subsequently well. A diagnosis of TGA had been made. He had no further amnesic episodes or memory issues until the onset of his progressive memory problems seven years later, which was felt to be entirely distinct from his previous episode of TGA.

Case Study 6.2: Subjective Memory Complaint Subsequent, but not Consequent, to TGA?
A 72-year-old academic complained of difficulties recalling peoples' names and their associations, perhaps dating back a couple of years. Her concerns stemmed in part from the family history of Alzheimer's disease in her mother with onset in her late 70s. Furthermore, the patient had had an episode of

transient global amnesia for which she had been briefly hospitalised some nine years earlier. She reported that brain imaging had not been undertaken at that time, but pursuing the clinical records proved this not to be the case (presumably a reflection of her acute amnesic state), she had had a CT brain scan which was normal. She now scored at ceiling on both the Montreal Cognitive Assessment and the Mini-Addenbrooke's Cognitive Examination.

However, since TGA likely represents functional change in the hippocampus (Sect. 9.7), as suggested by diffusion-weighted magnetic resonance imaging (Sect. 5.1.2), is it possible that TGA might predispose to future hippocampal pathology?

Nausieda and Sherman reported dementia in 6% of 32 TGA patients followed up for 3 years [9]. Gandolfo et al. reported only 3 of 102 TGA patients with intellectual deterioration in a prospectively identified group followed up for a mean of 82 months [4].

One study has suggested that TGA may be a risk factor for the syndrome of mild cognitive impairment (MCI). Although MCI has been variously defined, it may represent a prodromal phase of dementing disorder, most frequently Alzheimer's disease. Borroni et al. undertook neuropsychological assessment in 55 TGA patients at least one year after the attack and also in 80 age-matched controls, finding worse performance on tests evaluating verbal and non-verbal long-term memory and attention in the former group but with comparable global cognitive functions [1]. Applying then current criteria for amnestic MCI (aMCI; [75]), nearly one-third of the TGA subjects (18/55 = 32.7%) fulfilled the criteria. It was concluded that objective memory deficits fulfilling aMCI criteria may persist over time in TGA patients [1]. To my knowledge, no subsequent study has been reported which corroborates this finding.

Arena et al. followed up 221 TGA cases for a mean of 12 years and found no evidence of increased risk of subsequent cognitive impairment compared to a matched control group [76].

The systematic review of long-term TGA prognosis reported by Liampas et al. found contradictory results for dementia, with evidence for both a similar and increased risk compared to healthy controls [14]. Hence, the issue of long-term cognitive outcome in TGA requires further long-term follow-up studies in large cohorts, which might also profitably address whether or not cognitive outcomes differ between patients with single-episode and recurrent TGA.

6.3.2 Cognitive Decline: Progressive Aphasia

Graff-Radford and Josephs reported three patients diagnosed with primary progressive aphasia (PPA) who had had episodes of TGA prior to their presentation with linguistic problems and speculated that the conditions might be related [77]. Of possible relevance, all three patients had recurrent attacks of TGA (Sect. 6.2.2). This paper prompted a response from Nitrini and colleagues [78] drawing attention to an abstract they had published some years previously describing two patients with the semantic variant of PPA (or semantic dementia) who had both had recurrent episodes of TGA prior to the development of aphasia, in one case predating it by 7 and 6 years ([79], p.332, Abstract 34). I am not aware of any further publications on this possible association and have not observed it in any patient in my TGA case series, or examples of prior TGA in patients with progressive aphasia syndromes. Hence, Glannon's assertion that "a significant number of people diagnosed with TGA … have been subsequently diagnosed with primary progressive aphasia" ([80], p.64) does not currently bear scrutiny.

6.3.3   Stroke

In light of the generally favourable vascular risk factor profile in TGA patients as compared to TIA patients (Sect. 7.11), future stroke risk in TGA patients may be anticipated to be low. Miller et al. found no increased risk for subsequent stroke in their report of 277 TGA patients with average follow-up of 80 months [7]. Gandolfo et al. reported only four instances of stroke in 102 TGA patients identified in a prospective study and followed up for a mean of 82 months [4]. Hodges [22] and Pantoni et al. [10] found a lower risk of stroke at follow-up in TGA compared to TIA patients. Arena et al. [76] found no evidence of increased risk of subsequent cerebrovascular events in 221 TGA patients followed up for a mean of 12 years in comparison with a matched control group. The systematic review of TGA prognosis by Liampas et al. found similar vascular (and mortality) risks in TGA and healthy controls [14]. Of course, these reassuring data do not obviate addressing vascular risk factors in TGA patients should they be identified.

Recently, however, a propensity-matched cohort study from Korea (>10,000 patients) has suggested an increased risk [81], in direct contradiction to the findings of another propensity-matched study from the USA (>21,000 patients) [82]. Attempting to explain these differences, Romoli and Muccioli noted the increased frequency of cardiovascular risk factors in the American population and the female predominance in the Korean cohort, with risk emerging over longer follow-up [83]. This subject area remains one of active research.

6.3.4   Epilepsy

The Oxford TGA study reported that 7% of patients with apparent TGA subsequently developed epilepsy, usually of complex partial type ([22], p.41,46–7,56,121,123,124–5137). This suggested to the investigators that the original "TGA" attacks were in fact due to seizures. Another possible explanation is that TGA attacks may predispose to epileptic attacks as a consequence of microstructural damage to the hippocampus (Sect. 3.2.2). The occasional emergence of TEA in patients with prior episodes of TGA (Sect. 3.2.2) might also be pertinent to this argument.

Although the case–control study of Arena et al. did not suggest any increased risk of subsequent epileptic seizures in TGA patients followed up for a mean of 12 years [76], a population-based cohort study has reported an association of TGA with increased long-term risk of epilepsy. The adjusted hazard ratio for epilepsy in TGA cohorts was 6.50 (95% confidence interval 1.87–22.68, $p = 0.003$) compared with non-TGA cohorts after adjusting for age, gender and comorbidities [84]. A systematic review of long-term TGA prognosis could not exclude an increased risk of epilepsy in TGA patients [14].

6.3.5 Depression

The finding of depression as a risk factor for recurrent TGA [61, 62] was previously mentioned. In a population-based cohort study, Hsieh et al. found no increase in the long-term risk of depression in TGA patients versus matched non-TGA subjects (adjusted hazard ratio 1.67; 95% confidence interval 0.85–3.25, $p = 0.139$) [85]. Whilst TGA patients may have anxious personality traits (Sect. 7.10) and experience depressive mood during an attack (Sect. 2.1.2), long-term risk for depression does not appear to be increased.

6.4 Management

Once the diagnosis of TGA has been established, there is no specific treatment other than patient explanation and reassurance. As TGA episodes are self-limiting, there is no indication for acute medication.

Future management is expectant, since there is currently no compelling evidence of increased risk of future stroke, epilepsy or other cognitive impairments (see Sect. 6.3). No specific lifestyle advice is indicated, unless attacks have come on during specific activities (e.g. exercise) which might be avoided or moderated.

6.4.1 Driving

A particular management issue relates to driving after TGA. Advice to stop driving is not infrequently issued by clinicians unfamiliar with TGA who encounter these patients, probably because of concerns about stroke and epilepsy [86].

Different jurisdictions have different rules relating to fitness to drive, which should be consulted and adhered to. In the United Kingdom, the Driver and Vehicle Licencing Authority (DVLA) has placed no restriction on driving following a single episode of TGA, and there is no statutory obligation to inform DVLA following a single episode [87], and this remains the case at time of writing (31/12/2021). This contrasts with previous DVLA recommendations, prior to 1991, in which TGA was regarded as equivalent to TIA and driving for 3 months was not permitted ([22], p.59).

Reports of patients driving safely over long distances during attacks of TGA (e.g. [88, 89].), sometimes referred to as the "unconscious driving phenomenon" (see Case Study 3.3), may be taken to indicate that driving skills, an aspect of procedural memory, are not impaired. Memory impairment does not necessarily impair most aspects of driving performance, as shown by a study of two experienced drivers with bilateral hippocampal lesions causing severe amnesia [90].

6.4.2   Pharmacotherapy

The low recurrence rate of TGA, meaning that most patients suffer only a single attack, currently obviates routine prophylactic treatment, although one report claiming successful prophylaxis with a beta-blocker, metoprolol, has appeared [91]. Recurrent-TGA attacks following withdrawal and change of beta-blocker therapy for migraine has also been reported [70]. In a patient reported to have 5–6 TGA attacks per year during attacks of migraine without aura, verapamil and valproate were said to reduce the frequency of TGA [72].

It may be that those with recurrent TGA do require more than simple reassurance, but further studies will be required to address this question.

6.5   Summary and Recommendations

Generally, TGA is a benign condition and patients can be reassured about long-term outcome. Nevertheless, some deficits in verbal memory, beyond the amnesia for the attack itself, and in spatial navigation may persist although the practical consequences seem to be few. Long-term risk of dementia remains uncertain. There is a distinct but low recurrence rate for TGA to which migraine may predispose. Some patients may develop partial epilepsy but whether this reflects initial misdiagnosis or the consequence of TGA remains to be fully defined. Further studies focussing particularly on outcome in patients with recurrent TGA are required.

References

1. Borroni B, Agosti C, Brambilla C, et al. Is transient global amnesia a risk factor for amnestic mild cognitive impairment? J Neurol. 2004;251:1125–7.
2. Chen ST, Tang LM, Hsu WC, Lee TH, Ro LS, Wu YR. Clinical features, vascular risk factors, and prognosis for transient global amnesia in Chinese patients. J Stroke Cerebrovasc Dis. 1999;8:295–9.

3. Colombo A, Scarpa M. Transient global amnesia: pathogenesis and prognosis. Eur Neurol. 1988;28:111–4.
4. Gandolfo C, Caponnetto C, Conti M, Dagnino N, Del Sette M, Primavera A. Prognosis of transient global amnesia: a long-term follow-up study. Eur Neurol. 1992;32:52–7.
5. Hinge HH, Jensen TS, Kjaer M, Marquardsen J, de Fine OB. The prognosis of transient global amnesia. Results of a multicenter study. Arch Neurol. 1986;43:673–6.
6. Jensen TS, de Fine OB. Transient global amnesia—its clinical and pathophysiological basis and prognosis. Acta Neurol Scand. 1981;63:220–30.
7. Miller JW, Petersen RC, Metter EJ, Millikan CH, Yanagihara T. Transient global amnesia: clinical characteristics and prognosis. Neurology. 1987;37:733–7.
8. Mueller HR. Transient global amnesia. With a contribution to its prognosis [in German]. Schweiz Rundsch Med Prax. 1989;78:970–5.
9. Nausieda PA, Sherman IV. Long-term prognosis in transient global amnesia. JAMA. 1979;241:392–3.
10. Pantoni L, Bertini E, Lamassa M, Pracucci G, Inzitari D. Clinical features, risk factors, and prognosis in transient global amnesia: a follow-up study. Eur J Neurol. 2005;12:350–6.
11. Romoli M, Tuna MA, Li L, et al. Time trends, frequency, characteristics and prognosis of short-duration transient global amnesia. Eur J Neurol. 2020;27:887–93.
12. Uttner I, Weber S, Freund W, Schmitz B, Ramspott M, Huber R. Transient global amnesia – full recovery without persistent cognitive impairment. Eur Neurol. 2007;58:146–51.
13. Uttner I, Prexl S, Freund W, Unrath A, Bengel D, Huber R. Long-term outcome in transient global amnesia patients with and without hyperintensities in the CA1 region of the hippocampus. Eur Neurol. 2012;67:155–60.
14. Liampas I, Raptopoulou M, Siokas V, et al. The long-term prognosis of transient global amnesia: a systematic review. Rev Neurosci. 2021;32:531–43.
15. Guillery-Girard B, Desgranges B, Urban C, Piolino P, de la Sayette V, Eustache F. The dynamic time course of memory recovery in transient global amnesia. J Neurol Neurosurg Psychiatry. 2004;75:1532–40.
16. Kapur N, Millar J, Abbott P, Carter M. Recovery of function processes in human amnesia: evidence from transient global amnesia. Neuropsychologia. 1998;36:99–107.
17. Roman-Campos G, Poser CM, Wood FB. Persistent retrograde memory deficit after transient global amnesia. Cortex. 1980;16:509–18.
18. Mazzucchi A, Moretti G, Caffarra P, Parma M. Neuropsychological functions in the follow-up of transient global amnesia. Brain. 1980;103:161–78.
19. Cattaino G, Querin F, Pomes A, Piazza P. Transient global amnesia. Acta Neurol Scand. 1984;70:385–90.
20. Daniel BT. Transient global amnesia. Print version and ebook: Amazon; 2012.
21. Hodges JR, Oxbury SM. Persistent memory impairment following transient global amnesia. J Clin Exp Neuropsychol. 1990;12:904–20.
22. Hodges JR. Transient amnesia. Clinical and neuropsychological aspects. London: WB Saunders; 1991.
23. Le Pira F, Giuffrida S, Maci T, Reggio E, Zappala G, Perciavalle V. Cognitive findings after transient global amnesia: role of prefrontal cortex. Appl Neuropsychol. 2005;12:212–7.
24. Guillery-Girard B, Quinette P, Desgranges B, et al. Long-term memory following transient global amnesia: an investigation of episodic and semantic memory. Acta Neurol Scand. 2006;114:329–33.
25. Jäger T, Szabo K, Griebe M, Bazner H, Moller H, Hennerici MG. Selective disruption of hippocampus-mediated recognition memory processes after episodes of transient global amnesia. Neuropsychologia. 2009;47:70–6.
26. Noël A, Quinette P, Dayan J, et al. Influence of patients' emotional state on the recovery processes after a transient global amnesia. Cortex. 2011;47:981–91.
27. Schöberl F, Irving S, Pradhan C, et al. Prolonged allocentric navigation deficits indicate hippocampal damage in TGA. Neurology. 2019;92:e234–43.

28. Stracciari A, Lorusso S, Delli Ponti A, Mattarozzi K, Tempestini A. Cognitive functions after transient topographical amnesia. Eur J Neurol. 2002;9:401–5.
29. Naranjo-Fernandez C, Arjona A, Quiroga-Subirana P, et al. Transient topographical amnesia: a description of a series of eight case [in Spanish]. Rev Neurol. 2010;50:217–20.
30. Bender MB. Syndrome of isolated episode of confusion with amnesia. J Hillside Hosp. 1956;5:212–5.
31. Bender MB. Single episode of confusion with amnesia. Bull NY Acad Med. 1960;36:197–207.
32. Guyotat MM, Courjon J. Les ictus amnésiques. J Med Lyon. 1956;37:697–701.
33. Fisher CM, Adams RD. Transient global amnesia. Acta Neurol Scand. 1964;40(Suppl9):1–81.
34. Lou H. Repeated episodes of transient global amnesia. Acta Neurol Scand. 1968;44:612–8.
35. Hodges JR, Warlow CP. Syndromes of transient amnesia: towards a classification. A study of 153 cases. J Neurol Neurosurg Psychiatry. 1990;53:834–43.
36. Bermejo PE, García-Cobos E. Recurrent post-coital transient global amnesia. Rev Neurol. 2010;51:316–7.
37. Gonzalez-Martinez V, Comte F, de Verbizier D, Carlander B. Transient global amnesia: concordant hippocampal abnormalities on positron emission tomography and magnetic resonance imaging. Arch Neurol. 2010;67:510–1.
38. Lane RJ. Recurrent coital amnesia. J Neurol Neurosurg Psychiatry. 1997;63:260.
39. Bucuk M, Tomic Z, Tuskan-Mohar L, Bonifacic D, Bralic M, Jurjevic A. Recurrent transient global amnesia at high altitude. High Alt Med Biol. 2008;9:239–40.
40. Schakelaar JH. Two attacks of transient global amnesia within a year: a case report. Cases J. 2009;2:6309.
41. Stracciari A, Lorusso S, Pazzaglia P. Transient topographical amnesia. J Neurol Neurosurg Psychiatry. 1994;57:1423–5.
42. Shindo A, Satoh M, Kajikawa H, Ito N, Miyamura H, Tomimoto H. Recurrent transient topographical amnesia: a patient with frequent episodes. J Neurol. 2011;258:1566–7.
43. Toledo M, Pujadas F, Purroy F, Lara N, Quintana M, Alvarez-Sabin J. Recurrent transient global amnesia, a manifestation of ischemic cerebrovascular disease [in Spanish]. Med Clin (Barc). 2005;125:361–5. [Erratum Med Clin (Barc). 2006;126:316]
44. Quinette P, Guillery-Girard B, Dayan J, de la Sayette V, Marquis S, Viader F, Desgranges B, Eustache F. What does transient global amnesia really mean? Review of the literature and thorough study of 142 cases. Brain. 2006;129:1640–58.
45. Brigo F, Tezzon F, Nardone R. "Once again she forgets everything!": a patient with four episodes of transient global amnesia within less than 5 years. Acta Neurol Belg. 2018;118:319–20.
46. Rumpl E, Rumpl H. Recurrent transient global amnesia in a case with cerebrovascular lesions and livedo reticularis (Sneddon syndrome). J Neurol. 1979;221:127–31.
47. Grande LA, Loeser JD, Samil A. Recurrent transient global amnesia with intrathecal baclofen. Anesth Analg. 2008;106:1284–7.
48. Sealove BA, Aledort LM, Stacy CB, Halperin JL. Recurrent orthostatic global amnesia in a patient with postoperative hyperfibrinogenemia. J Stroke Cerebrovasc Dis. 2008;17:241–3.
49. Tassinari CA, Ciarmatori C, Alesi C, et al. Transient global amnesia as a postictal state from recurrent partial seizures. Epilepsia. 1991;32:882–5.
50. Melo TP, Ferro JM, Paiva T. Are brief or recurrent transient global amnesias of epileptic origin? J Neurol Neurosurg Psychiatry. 1994;57:622–5.
51. Gallassi R, Stracciari A, Morreale A, Lorusso S, Rebucci GG, Lugaresi E. Transient global amnesia: neuropsychological findings after single and multiple attacks. Neurol. 1993;33:294–8.
52. Lampl Y, Sadeh M, Lorberboym M. Transient global amnesia—not always a benign process. Acta Neurol Scand. 2004;110:75–9.
53. Toledo M, Pujadas F, Grivé E, Alvarez-Sabin J, Quintana M, Rovira A. Lack of evidence for arterial ischemia in transient global amnesia. Stroke. 2008;39:476–9.
54. Agosti C, Akkawi NM, Borroni B, Padovani A. Recurrency in transient global amnesia: a retrospective study. Eur J Neurol. 2006;13:986–9.

55. Auyeung M, Tsoi TH, Cheung CM, et al. Association of diffusion weighted imaging abnormalities and recurrence in transient global amnesia. J Clin Neurosci. 2011;18:531–4.
56. Moon Y, Moon WJ, Han SH. The structural connectivity of the recurrent transient global amnesia. Acta Neurol Scand. 2016;134:160–4.
57. Kim J, Lee DA, Kim HC, Lee H, Park KM. Brain networks in patients with isolated or recurrent transient global amnesia. Acta Neurol Scand. 2021;144:465–73.
58. Lee DA, Lee S, Kim DW, Lee H, Park KM. Effective connectivity alteration according to recurrence in transient global amnesia. Neuroradiology. 2021;63:1441–9.
59. Morris KA, Rabinstein AA, Young NP. Factors associated with risk of recurrent transient global amnesia. JAMA Neurol. 2020;77:1551–8.
60. Alessandro L, Calandri IL, Fernandez Suarez M, et al. Transient global amnesia: clinical features and prognostic factors suggesting recurrence. Arq Neuropsiquiatr. 2019;77:3–9.
61. Tynas R, Panegyres PK. Factors determining recurrence in transient global amnesia. BMC Neurol. 2020;20:83.
62. Oliveira R, Teodoro T, Marques IB. Risk factors predicting recurrence of transient global amnesia. Neurol Sci. 2021;42:2039–43.
63. Ganeshan R, Betz M, Scheitz JF, et al. Frequency of silent brain infarction in transient global amnesia. J Neurol. 2022;269:1422–6.
64. Liampas I, Raptopoulou M, Mpourlios S, et al. Factors associated with recurrent transient global amnesia: systematic review and pathophysiological insights. Rev Neurosci. 2021;32:751–65.
65. Larner AJ. Recurrent transient global amnesia: Is there a link to familial history? Prog Neurol Psychiatry. 2017;21(4):17–9.
66. Larner AJ. Recurrent TGA: link to family history? Prog Neurol Psychiatry. 2018;22(1):18.
67. Corston RN, Godwin-Austen RB. Transient global amnesia in four brothers. J Neurol Neurosurg Psychiatry. 1982;45:375–7.
68. Munro JM, Loizou LA. Transient global amnesia—familial incidence. J Neurol Neurosurg Psychiatry. 1982;45:1070.
69. Dupuis MM, Pierre PH, Gonsette RE. Transient global amnesia and migraine in twin sisters. J Neurol Neurosurg Psychiatry. 1987;50:816–7.
70. Vyhnalek M, Bojar M, Jerabek J, Hort J. Long lasting recurrent familiar [sic] transient global amnesia after betablocker withdrawal: case report. Neuro Endocrinol Lett. 2008;29:44–6.
71. Segers-van Rijn J, de Bruijn SFTM. Transient global amnesia: a genetic disorder? Eur Neurol. 2010;63:186–7.
72. Maggioni F, Mainardi F, Bellamio M, Zanchin G. Transient global amnesia triggered by migraine in monozygotic twins. Headache. 2011;51:1305–8.
73. Dupuis M, Vandeponseele M, Jacquerye P, et al. Familial transient global amnesia: report of 10 families. J Neurol Sci. 2017;381(Suppl):381.
74. Daniel ES. Early diagnosis and treatment of dementia presenting as transient global amnesia in a 76-year-old man. Prim Care Companion J Clin Psychiatry. 2004;6:248–51.
75. Petersen RC, Smith GE, Waring SC, Ivnik RJ, Tangalos EG, Kokmen E. Mild cognitive impairment: clinical characterization and outcome. Arch Neurol. 1999;56:303–8. [Erratum Arch Neurol. 1999;56:760]
76. Arena JE, Brown RD, Mandrekar J, Rabinstein AA. Long-term outcome in patients with transient global amnesia: a population-based study. Mayo Clin Proc. 2017;92:399–405.
77. Graff-Radford J, Josephs KA. Primary progressive aphasia and transient global amnesia. Arch Neurol. 2012;69:401–4.
78. Nitrini R, Hosogi-Senaha ML, Carmelli P. Primary progressive aphasia and transient global amnesia. Arch Neurol. 2012;69:1214.
79. [No authors listed]Abstracts first Brazilian symposium of frontotemporal lobar degeneration. Dement Neuropsychol. 2007;1:320–32.

80. Glannon W. The neuroethics of memory. From total recall to oblivion. Cambridge: Cambridge University Press; 2019.
81. Lee SH, Kim KY, Lee JW, Park SJ, Jung JM. Risk of ischaemic stroke in patients with transient global amnesia: a propensity-matched cohort study. Stroke Vasc Neurol. 2021; https://doi.org/10.1136/svn-2021-001006. svn-2021-001006. Online ahead of print
82. Garg A, Limaye K, Shaban A, Adams HP Jr, Leira EC. Transient global amnesia does not increase the risk of subsequent ischemic stroke: a propensity score-matched analysis. J Neurol. 2021;268:3301–6.
83. Romoli M, Muccioloi L. Transient global amnesia and stroke: not that benign? Stroke Vasc Neurol. 2021; https://doi.org/10.1136/svn-2021-0011384. svn-2021-0011384 Online ahead of print
84. Hsieh SW, Yang YH, Ho BL, Yang ST, Chen CH. The long-term risk of epilepsy after transient global amnesia: a population-based cohort study. Clin Neurol Neurosurg. 2020;197:106086.
85. Hsieh SW, Chen CH, Ho B, Yang ST, Yang YH. Long-term risk of depression after transient global amnesia: a population-based study. Psychiatry Clin Neurosci. 2020;74:413–4.
86. Larner AJ. Transient global amnesia in the district general hospital. Int J Clin Pract. 2007;61:255–8.
87. Cartlidge NE. Transient global amnesia. BMJ. 1991;302:62–3.
88. Gordon B, Marin O. Transient global amnesia: an extensive case report. J Neurol Neurosurg Psychiatry. 1979;42:572–5.
89. Huang CF, Pai MC. Transient amnesia in a patient with left temporal tumor. Symptomatic transient global amnesia or an epileptic amnesia? Neurologist. 2008;14:196–200.
90. Anderson SW, Rizzo M, Skaar N, et al. Amnesia and driving. J Clin Exp Neuropsychol. 2007;29:1–12.
91. Berlit P. Successful prophylaxis of recurrent transient global amnesia with metoprolol. Neurology. 2000;55:1937–8.

Chapter 7
Epidemiology of TGA (1): Possible Predisposing Factors

Abstract This chapter examines factors identified in clinical and epidemiological studies as predisposing to episodes of TGA. None of these factors is either necessary or sufficient for the occurrence of TGA. Nevertheless, the more consistently implicated predisposing factors, such as a personal history of migraine, may give insights into disease pathogenesis. Precipitating factors for TGA are considered in the subsequent chapter.

Keywords TGA · Incidence · Predisposing factors

A number of factors have been described which though temporally remote from the onset of an attack of TGA may nevertheless predispose to it (i.e. increase the chance or risk of its occurrence). Of the reported predisposing or risk factors for TGA, some are more certain than others, based on the existing evidence.

7.1 Incidence

As a transient condition, of duration less than 24 h (if concordant with clinical diagnostic criteria [1] (see Table 2.1), no meaningful data on TGA prevalence can be collected, rather only incidence.

A limited number of studies of TGA incidence have been reported (Table 7.1) [2–10], most population-based [2–6, 8, 10] but some based on experience at a single centre [7, 9]. Annual incidence rates in these studies range between 2.9 and 12/100,000 of the population. The highest of these measures was recorded at Davos, Switzerland, located at relatively high altitude, prompting the suggestion that low temperature might contribute to TGA pathogenesis [9] (see Sect. 8.3). Govoni et al. noted a statistically significant difference in incidence rates with level of urbanisation and population density, prompting the suggestion that the stress related to urban living might contribute to pathogenesis [10] (see Sect. 7.10). Of course, one may

Table 7.1 Incidence studies of TGA

Reference	Study location	Annual incidence	Sex-specific incidence
Miller et al. (1987) [2]	Rochester, Minnesota, USA	5.2/100,000	–
Koski and Marttila (1990) [3]	Turku, Finland	10/100,000 (32/100,000 amongst those ≥50 years)	–
Hodges (1991) ([4], p.13)	Oxford, UK	3/100,000	–
Matias-Guiu et al. (1992) [5]	Alcoi, Spain	2.9/100,000	–
Lauria et al. (1997) [6]	Belluno, Italy	10.4/100,000 (crude); 8.6/100,000 (adjusted); 5.81/100,000 (retrospective study)	9.35/100,000 for men; 11.37/100,000 for women
Berli et al. (2009) [7]	Uster Hospital, Switzerland	6.8/100,000	–
Brigo et al. (2014) [8]	Merano, province of Bolzano, Italy	9.6/100,000 (crude); 6.4/100,000 (adjusted)	10.1/100,000 for men; 8.9/100,000 for women
Erba and Czaplinski (2017) [9]	Regional Hospital, Davos, Switzerland	12/100,000	–
Govoni et al. (2020) [10]	Ferrara, Italy	10.10/100,000 (crude)	8.40/100,000 for men; 11.60/100,000 for women

posit alternative explanations for these observations, such as underascertainment of cases in rural areas with less readily available access to medical services.

Only limited data on sex-specific incidence rates are available (Table 7.1), permitting no definitive conclusion as to whether this is greater in men or women. For example, the gender difference observed by Govoni et al. was not statistically significant [10].

7.2   Chronobiology: Time of Onset by Day, Month and Season

Quinette et al. reported a peak of TGA occurrence in spring and summer in their literature review (*n* = 46), but in their own cohort they found TGA episodes were distributed evenly throughout the year [11].

Keret et al. [12, 13] examined the seasonal incidence of TGA cases seen in a single tertiary care centre in Israel. Initially, they reported (in abstract) a series of 86 TGA patients (F:M = 54:32, 63% female; mean age 61 ± 10.3 years) seen over the period 2005–2013, in whom they found two incidence peaks, in November–December and in March [12]. In a later, substantive, paper, the time frame was broadened to 15 years (2000–2014), in which period 154 TGA patients were seen (F:M = 91:63, 59% female; mean age 62.8 ± 10.6 years), with incidence peaks in winter (December) and spring (March) [13]. The authors concluded that seasonal factors might contribute to TGA pathogenesis.

Govoni et al. found TGA cases to be evenly distributed by month and season in their incidence study [10].

Hoyer et al. [14] analysed data from two large TGA cohorts (n = 404 and 261, respectively) and found no variation of TGA occurrence by day of the week, month or season of the year, in contrast to a robust circadian rhythm of incidence (mid-morning, late afternoon) (Sect. 2.1.3).

In the author's series, TGA seasonal incidence has been examined in two ways: by meteorological season (for the northern hemisphere: Spring = March–May; Summer = June–August; Autumn = September–November; Winter = December–February) and by quarter of the year (Q1 = January–March; Q2 = April–June; Q3 = July–September; Q4 = October–December) approximating to the astronomical seasons, defined by the solstices and equinoxes, as in the Gregorian calendar (Fig. 7.1a, b respectively; updated from [15, 16]). The null hypothesis that cases did not differ by either season or quarter was not rejected.

Rather than season per se, ambient temperature might be a predisposing and/or precipitating (see Sect. 8.3) factor for TGA. One study suggested an association between TGA occurrence and low ambient temperature [17]. Cases of TGA related to high altitude [9] might also reflect a relationship to ambient temperature.

7.3   Place of Onset: Geographical Distribution

Cases of TGA have been reported from all the inhabited continents of the world, even remote locations such as Polynesia [18]. There do not appear to be any geographical "hot-spots" of high incidence, but to the author's knowledge, no systematic study of population-based prevalence has been undertaken.

It has been reported that TGA (and migraine) is more common in Latin American patients with the antiphospholipid syndrome (APS+) than in European APS+ patients [19].

7.4   Patient Age

Most studies find that TGA is typically a condition of mid-life, particularly affecting those in their 50s and 60s, and distinctly unusual at earlier ages (<40 years; Table 7.2).

In the survey of the author's experience (n = 50), median patient age was 64.8 years (Fig. 7.2). Those acute amnesic patients excluded for not conforming to

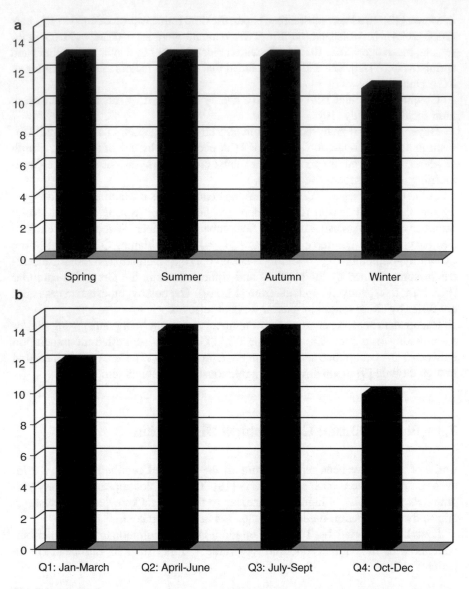

Fig. 7.1 Distribution of consecutive cases fulfilling diagnostic criteria for TGA (*n* = 50) seen in author's clinic over 20-year period (2002–2021). (**a**) by meteorological season (Northern Hemisphere) of presentation (Spring = March–May; Summer = June–August; Autumn = September–November; Winter = December–February). (**b**) by quarter of presentation (Q1 = January–March; Q2 = April–June; Q3 = July–September; Q4 = October–December)

Hodges and Warlow's diagnostic criteria [1], and not definitely diagnosed with TEA based on Zeman's criteria [29], were slightly younger (median 62.2 years; Fig. 7.3). In the Oxford TGA study, non-TGA cases were non-significantly younger than definite TGA cases (mean age 60.8 vs 62.3 years) ([4], p.113–4, Fig. A.2).

Table 7.2 Age and gender of TGA patients (selected reports)

Reference	N	Age (years)	Gender
Hodges and Warlow (1990) [1]	114 prospective, single clinic (UK)	62.3 ± 8.5 (range 35–85)	66% male
Hodges and Warlow (1990) [1]	752 literature review	61.2 (range 20–92)	53% male
Quinette et al. (2006) [11]	142 prospective, single clinic (France)	63.9 ± 8.3 (range 32–81)	33.1% male
Quinette et al. (2006) [11]	246 (age) 1333 (gender) literature review	60.3 ± 9.6 (range 21–85)	46.4% male
Berli et al. (2009) [7]	20 retrospective, single centre (Switzerland)	67 ± 7.3 (range 58–86)	60% female
Agosti et al. (2010) [20]	243 consecutive enrolment, 2 hospitals (Italy and Lebanon)	64.0 ± 8.3	44.9% female
Ahn et al. (2011) [21]	203 retrospective, single centre (South Korea)	60.1 ± 9.3	41.4% male
Ryoo et al. (2012) [22]	73 single centre (South Korea)	59.7 ± 9.5 (range 43–76)	72.6% female
Döhring et al. (2014) [23]	113 single centre (Germany)	65.4 ± 7.6	54.9% female
Keret et al. (2016) [13]	154 retrospective, hospital data (Israel)	62.8 ± 10.6	41% male
Arena et al. (2017) [24]	221 epidemiology database for single county (USA)	65.6 ± 12.2	50.2% female
Alessandro et al. (2019) [25]	203 single centre (Argentina)	65 (20–84)	52% female
Higashida et al. (2020) [26]	261 databases of four medical centres (Japan)	65.3 ± 8.6	61% female
Morris et al. (2020) [27]	1044 retrospective, single centre (USA)	75.0 ± 11.5	55.1% male
Szabo et al. (2020) [28]	390 prospective, single centre (Germany)	66.1 ± 7.8 (range 37–86)	39.5% male
Larner (2022)	50 prospective, single clinic (UK)	64.8 ± 6.9 (range 47–78)	58% female

Fig. 7.2 Age and gender distribution of consecutive cases fulfilling diagnostic criteria for TGA ($n = 50$) seen in author's clinic over 20-year period (2002–2021)

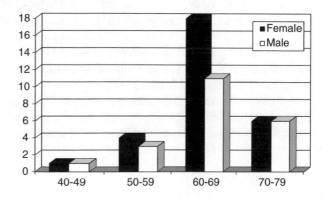

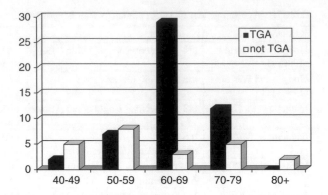

Fig. 7.3 Age distribution of consecutive cases of transient amnesia fulfilling ($n = 50$) and not fulfilling ($n = 23$) diagnostic criteria for TGA seen in author's clinic over 20-year period (2002–2021)

Although cases of TGA have been reported in young people (e.g. [30–35]), these are rare, and some predate diagnostic criteria so that caveats about the diagnosis apply (Sect. 1.3 and Sect. 2.2.2). Some have occurred in the context of exercise [33, 35], others in the context of migraine [30, 35]. An adolescent with two episodes labelled as TGA precipitated by emotion had temporal and occipital lobe embolic infarction in the context of congenital heart disease [34], raising the possibility of epileptic events. Certainly, the differential diagnosis requires careful consideration in patients under 40 years of age who are suspected of having TGA, and should include the possibility of acute confusional migraine [36] (Sect. 3.4.1; Case Study 3.3).

Cases of TGA are rarely reported in the oldest old people (>80 years). It is not clear whether this is simply underascertainment, against the background of the increasing prevalence of memory disorders in older people, or whether the elderly oldest old people are in some way protected from TGA, mechanism(s) unknown (see Sects. 9.4 and 9.7.6).

7.5   Patient Gender

The precise distribution of TGA by gender is uncertain, with different findings in different studies (Table 7.2). For example, in Hodges and Warlow's series of 114 patients, males outnumbered females [1], whereas Quinette et al. found no significant gender difference when pooling 1333 patients reported in 52 published case studies and 34 group studies (46.4% male, 53.6% women; $\chi 2 = 0.48$; df $= 1$; $p = 0.49$), although in their own series of 142 cases there was a 2:1 F:M preponderance (66.9% female, 33.1% male) [11].

A four-year survey (2002–2005 inclusive) of the author's practice [37] identified eight cases fulfilling diagnostic criteria for TGA, all of whom were female (age range 48–71 years). The preponderance of female cases was confirmed when the survey was extended to 6 years (F:M = 10:1 = 91% female) [38], 9 years (F:M = 11:5 = 69%) [39], 12 years (F:M = 14:10 = 58%) [40], 15 years (F:M = 20:14 = 59%) ([16], p.99), and at 20 years, the ratio was F:M = 29:21 (= 58%; Fig. 7.2). The falling ratio may indicate that the initial female preponderance was simply a chance observation associated with the small number of cases seen.

7.6 Patient Ethnicity

There do not seem to be any studies specifically addressing the role of patient ethnicity in the pathogenesis of TGA. It has certainly been reported from around the world, including relative geographical isolates such as Polynesia [18]. A nationwide inpatient sample analysis from the USA, including nearly 50,000 TGA patients, explored race-specific variables associated with TGA and reported that the odds of being diagnosed with TGA was lower for African Americans, Hispanics and Asians/others compared to Whites [41].

7.7 Patient Social Class

Hodges found no definite evidence of differences in TGA cases according to social class, although there was a non-significant difference in the proportion of patients from social class I ([4], p.15).

7.8 Family History of TGA

TGA has generally been considered as a sporadic condition. Although there is no suggestion that it has a monogenic Mendelian pattern of inheritance, nevertheless occasional familial clusters have been reported in the literature (Table 7.3). Hodges and Warlow suggested that the overall rate of familial TGA in their series was 1.75% (95% confidence interval = 0%–4.2%) [1].

Most familial reports have involved siblings (Table 7.3; Case Study 7.1), with two sets of twins (one monozygotic [51], the other probably so [45]), with only occasional definite [43, 47, 49, 57] or possible [1, 48, 56] instances of parental involvement. Only one account of familial involvement with more distant relatives, specifically a proband whose two aunts were apparently affected [52], has been found.

Case Study 7.1: Family History of TGA

Following a previous publication on the subject of familial TGA [56], the author was contacted by a family from western Canada with a family history of TGA. A 61-year-old woman had an episode of amnesia following a bike ride and during a period of emotional stress. Features were typical for TGA. CT brain scan and CT angiogram of the circle of Willis performed on the same day were both normal. There was no recurrence over the next five years. However, at that time her 60-year-old brother had an episode of TGA. After skiing, he took a chairlift to ascend, but on getting off had no recollection of the ride up or where he was. He knew who he was but had no understanding of why he was on a mountain. He repeatedly asked where his wife was. From the time on the chair lift to when he started to retain short-term memory was approximately 1 hour. There was no personal or family history of migraine.

Table 7.3 Reports of familial cases of TGA and their history of migraine (adapted and updated from [16], p.100–1) (see Table 6.2 for reports of recurrent TGA in these cases)

Reference	TGA patient details	Migraine history
Corston and Godwin-Austen (1982) [42]	Four male siblings, 2–3 attacks each, when aged in 60s and 70s. Three-fourth had TGA attacks in context of exercise	None
Munro and Loizou (1982) [43]	Two siblings (F:M) and their father, one to three attacks in 50s to 60s	Not commented on
Stracciari and Rebucci (1986) [44]	Two siblings (F:M), attacks in 70s and 50s respectively, latter associated with exercise on a windy day	Both had prior history of migraine, F until menopause, M in adolescence
Dupuis et al. (1987) [45]	Twin sisters (probably monozygotic), attacks (2 and 1, respectively) in 60s	Both migraineurs since adolescence; both attacks in first sister followed by severe migraine
Hodges and Warlow (1990) [1]	60-year-old man; sister, mother, also affected. 66-year-old woman; brother also affected	Not specifically commented on
Agosti et al. (2007) [46]	Three female siblings in their 60s, attacks following emotional upset, cold shower and sexual intercourse, respectively	Not commented on
Vyhnalek et al. (2008) [47]	Male, 2 episodes aged 52, 54. Father 1 episode aged 50; sister 1 episode aged 52	Proband had migraine without aura from adolescence; no migraine in father or sister
Segers-van Rijn and de Bruijn (2010) [48]	Four siblings (3F:1M) and possibly their mother, attacks after exercise (3) and air travel (1), and on birthday; attacks between 50s and 70s	One of the female siblings had history of migraine with aura

Table 7.3 (continued)

Reference	TGA patient details	Migraine history
Galovic et al. (2011) (abstract only) [49]	4 siblings and their mother; AAO ca. 70 years, all single episodes, several associated with Valsalva manoeuvres	Not commented on
Goossens et al. (2011) (abstract only) [50]	Two sisters, attacks at age 61 and 57, respectively	Both had migraine with aura from adolescence; elder had headache at time of TGA
Maggioni et al. (2011) [51]	Two monozygotic twin brothers aged 50 and 49 at onset	Elder had 5–6 attacks per year during migraine without aura (MO) attacks, frequency reduced by verapamil and valproate; younger had 4 episodes all during MO
Davies and Larner (2012) [52]	Female and two maternal aunts, attacks in 50s and/or 60s, after exercise in the index case	Migraine in index case, no information on other cases
Dupuis et al. (2013) (abstract only) [53]	7 families	No other details available from published abstract
Dandapat et al. (2015) [54]	Two sisters, age 57 (precipitated by sex) and 71	No history of migraine; older sister had mild headache at time of TGA
Dupuis et al. (2017) (abstract only) [55]	10 families in cohort of 219 patients	History of migraine reported to be more frequent in familial cases
Larner (2017a) ([16], p.101) (personal communication; Case Study 7.1)	Two siblings (female aged 61, male aged 60), both associated with exercise	No history of migraine
Larner (2017b) [56]	Male, 2 episodes aged 61 and 64; father also reportedly had TGA, 2–3 episodes (uncertain)	No history of migraine
Larner (2017c) (unpublished, personal communication)	Two siblings (male aged 60, female aged 70), both associated with exercise	No history of migraine
Larner (2018) [57] (personal communication)	Two male siblings and their mother. Younger male sibling had three events, aged 60, 63, 66, first two after exercise (cycling)	No personal history of migraine in male with recurrent events
Larner (2018) [57] (personal communication)	Two female siblings. Younger female sibling had two events, aged 54 and 55, second after sexual activity. Older sibling had single event, aged 60, after sexual activity	Both siblings had history of migraine
Larner (2019a) (unpublished, personal communication)	Three siblings (1F:2M). Female 3 events aged 63, 68, 70, first after emotional upset, second after exercise. Single events in male siblings.	No personal history of migraine in female with recurrent events
Larner (2019b) (unpublished, personal communication)	Two siblings (1F:1M). Female 67, male 55, both exercise associated (gardening, running).	Female 2 or 3 migraines about 30 years earlier; male 1 migraine 25–30 years earlier
Larner (2019c) (unpublished, personal communication)	Two female siblings aged 79 and 75.	No history of migraine

Summing all these publications from which adequate information is available (hence excluding [49, 53, 55]), there were 53 patients from 21 families, with a slight female preponderance (F:M = 30:23, 57% female), with all TGA episodes occurring in the sixth to eighth decades of life (Table 7.3). Although details were incomplete, at least 16 (=30%) of these individuals had a history of migraine (11F:5M). Two (female) patients were reported to have had migraine-type headaches at the time of or immediately after TGA episodes [45, 50], and two monozygotic male twins had episodes during attacks of migraine without aura [51]. One man with a history of migraine without aura dating from adolescence had a first attack of TGA one month after withdrawal from a beta-blocker (atenolol) prescribed for hypertension for the previous 5 years [47].

Dupuis et al. [53] also examined the possibility of an hereditary aetiology for TGA. In a publication appearing in abstract only, they identified 9 families in the literature and 7 families "reported recently by one of us" (I have been unable to locate such a report, so presume it must have appeared in abstract only). Six of their personally observed families were from the same hospital and were compared to a database of 127 consecutive TGA patients. The 6 families were said to represent 4.7% of 127 TGA cases (with reported 95% CI 1.05%–8.45%), which seems to imply only 6 cases, so presumably the familial cases were by report rather than by direct observation.

References to the 9 families in the literature were not given, but I presume them to be those reported by Corston and Godwin-Austen [42], Munro and Loizou [43], Stracciari and Rebucci [44], Dupuis et al. [45], Hodges and Warlow ([1], 2 families), Agosti et al. [46], Segers-van Rijn and de Bruijn ([48]; co-authors on the abstract), and Goossens et al. ([50], co-authors on the abstract), but not those reported by Galovic et al. [49], as these were presented in abstract only, Vyhnalek et al. [47], as the title of this paper gives "familiar" rather than "familial" TGA, and perhaps Maggioni et al. [51], as too recent to be included. Summing all 16 families, Dupuis et al. reported 41 cases with mean age 61.8 years, 22 female (=53.7%), and 12 migrainous (=29.3%), with migraine and stress as "frequent risk factors". The familial cases were reported to be indistinguishable from sporadic cases [53].

Familial cases of transient epileptic amnesia (TEA; Sect. 3.2) have rarely been reported, and never, to my knowledge, in a substantive paper [58, 59].

Possible genetic contributions to the pathogenesis of TGA are discussed in Sects. 9.5 and 9.7.

7.9 Migraine

Migraine may be a symptomatic cause of amnesia, which enters the differential diagnosis of TGA (Sect. 3.4.1; Table 3.2). This may require particular consideration in young people with attacks purported to be TGA (for example, acute confusional migraine; Sect. 7.4). Migraine might also be considered as a precipitating factor for TGA (Sect. 8.6).

The possible association between TGA and migraine was recognised early in the history of TGA (Sect. 3.4.1): for example, Evans in 1966 reported two patients with attacks suggestive of TGA in the context of a history of migraine [60]. Other possible early reports include those of Frank (1976; amnesic episodes in migraine, "Migranedammerattacken", apparently identical with TGA) [61] and Caplan et al. in 1981 [62].

Migraine was more common in TGA patients than in both normal and TIA control subjects in the case–control study reported by Zorzon et al. [63]. A case–control study by Schmidtke and Ehmsen [64] showed a markedly increased prevalence of migraine in TGA patients and also of episodic tension-type headache. Quinette et al. used cluster hierarchical analysis of TGA cases to show that in younger patients a history of headache may be a risk factor for TGA [11]. Arena et al. followed up 221 TGA cases for a mean of 12 years and found that previous migraine was more common than in a matched control group [24].

A population-based cohort study from Taiwan found that migraine was associated with a higher risk of TGA. Over 150,000 migraine patients and their matched controls were followed up for a mean of 3 years, during which time the migraine cohort had a greater risk of developing TGA than the controls (7.59 vs 3.06/100,000 person-years, incidence rate ratio = 2.48). Female patients with migraine aged 40–60 years had a significantly higher risk of developing TGA (incidence rate ratio = 3.18). Incidence rates did not differ between migraine patients with or without aura [65].

In a nationwide inpatient sample analysis including nearly 50,000 TGA patients, patients with migraine were found to have a greater odds ratio (5.98, 95% CI 5.42–6.60) of having TGA [41].

A personal or family history of migraine is associated with, and may therefore be a risk factor for, recurrent TGA [25, 27, 66, 67]. A relationship to migraine might potentially explain a female preponderance of TGA cases, if such exists (Sect. 7.5), since migraine is more common in women. Many of the familial examples of TGA (Sect. 7.8) had migraine comorbidity (see Table 7.3).

The possible role of migraine in the pathogenesis of TGA is discussed in Sect. 9.4.

7.10   Patient Personality Traits and Psychological Factors

Acute TGA episodes may be associated with symptoms of anxiety and depression (Sect. 2.1.2) [68]), but whether these behavioural features are simply part of the acute phenomenology or reflect premorbid psychopathology or personality traits has been uncertain. Neri et al. found depressive symptoms, assessed by the Geriatric Depression Scale, in 8 of 20 TGA patients [69]. Inzitari et al. found that TGA patients scored higher on a scale that measured phobic attitudes than control patients with TIAs, suggesting that emotional arousal may be involved in TGA [70]. This may be consistent with the observation of emotional factors as precipitating factors of TGA (Sect. 8.1).

An increased frequency of personal and family history of psychiatric diseases was noted in TGA patients followed up for about 7 years and compared to TIA controls by Pantoni et al. [71]. Fischer et al. found indications of depressive disorders at the time of onset in 67.9% of a group of 28 TGA patients, compared to 12.5% in 25 TIA patients, prompting the authors to suggest that depressive disorders predispose to TGA, perhaps due to an imbalance in hippocampal neurotransmitters [72]. Quinette et al. found a past history of anxiety/depression in around 20% of the 129 patients in their personally observed series for whom this was investigated, and found a high frequency of psychological and emotional instability in TGA patients. They were of the view that TGA in women was associated with a history of anxiety and a pathological personality [11]. A study by Döhring et al. found a higher level of anxiety in patients who experienced a stress-related TGA precipitant compared to both those who did not and to controls, suggesting that increased susceptibility to psychological stress may be a risk factor for TGA [23].

The possibility that stress related to urban living might account for the differential incidence of TGA seen with level of urbanisation and population density [10] has been mentioned (Sect. 7.1), likewise that emotional stress might account for increased incidence of TGA following the onset of the COVID-19 pandemic [73] (Sect. 3.5.2).

7.11 Vascular Risk Factors and Stroke

Because of its sudden onset, the possibility that TGA may have a vascular aetiology has been considered from the time it was first described (Sect. 3.1). Transient ischaemic attack (TIA) and stroke enter the differential diagnosis of TGA (Sect. 3.1). Hence, the examination of vascular risk factors in TGA patients and comparison with TIA patients has been undertaken in a number of case–control studies.

The Oxford TGA study found no difference in the prevalence of vascular risk factors between prospectively identified TGA patients and matched controls, but significant differences with matched TIA controls ([4], p.125–32). In a prospective case–control study, Zorzon et al. found no evidence of increase in any vascular risk factor in 64 TGA patients compared with matched TIA patients and normal controls [63].

Retrospective studies have sometimes reached different conclusions. Hypertension was noted to be the most common vascular risk factor in one retrospective series of TGA cases (11/28) although no vascular risk factor was noted in about half of the cases [74]. Prevalence of vascular risk factors was found to be higher in TGA patients than healthy controls by Santos et al. [75]. A retrospective study of 131 TGA patients seen between 1993 and 2004 found a higher incidence of hypertension compared to 262 TIA patients, whereas diabetes mellitus, ischaemic heart disease and cerebrovascular disease were more common in the latter group [76]. In a cohort of TGA patients identified in the Framingham Heart Study, no significant differences were observed in the prevalence of vascular risk factors with a control group [77]. A retrospective case–control study of 293 TGA patients published by Jang et al. found a significantly higher prevalence of ischaemic heart disease and hyperlipidaemia than in TIA controls, although the latter had a higher prevalence of hypertension, diabetes mellitus, ischaemic stroke and atrial fibrillation. TGA patients also had a significantly higher prevalence of hyperlipidaemia, previous ischaemic stroke and ischaemic heart disease when compared to age- and sex-matched normal controls [78]. The difference between the findings of studies with prospective or retrospective design should be noted.

Tuduri et al. found no clinical differences between TGA patients with and without vascular risk factors [79]. Toledo et al. compared "unique-TGA" cases ($n = 98$) with "recurrent-TGA" cases ($n = 26$) and found that the latter had the same vascular risk factors as a comparison group of TIA patients. Furthermore, the recurrent-TGA patients had a significantly more frequent history of stroke and a trend to suffer new ischaemic events than patients in the unique-TGA group, prompting the suggestion that recurrent TGA be considered a manifestation of ischaemic cerebrovascular disease [80], but in a later study they appeared to revise their views [81] (see Sect. 6.2.2). Agosti et al. divided TGA patients ($n = 243$) according to whether or not they had evidence for internal jugular vein valve incompetence (IJVVI), a factor which might be relevant to TGA pathogenesis (Sect. 4.3.3.2 and Sect. 9.2.2). TGA patients with IJVVI showed a higher frequency of precipitating factors but had fewer vascular comorbidities than TGA patients without IJVVI, suggesting that different mechanisms might operate in individual episodes of TGA [20].

In a systematic review, Liampas et al. retrieved 23 observational studies from which they concluded that diabetes was protective for TGA, dyslipidaemia was not related, and only severe hypertension was associated [82]. Rogalewski et al. found that acute hypertensive peaks showed a strong association with TGA [83].

In conclusion, single episode TGA does not seem to share the same vascular risk factors as TIA but this might not necessarily be the case for recurrent episodes of TGA. The possible role of vascular pathology, arterial or venous, in the pathogenesis of TGA is considered in Sect. 9.2.

7.12 Structural Brain Lesions

Occasional reports associating TGA with the presence of a structural brain lesion have appeared. These most usually concern brain tumours, but even here the cases are rare, with one systematic review finding only about 20 cases [40] (Table 7.4). No cases of brain tumour were encountered in some large series (e.g. [1].). Agosti et al. would classify such patients as "TGA-b", in distinction from primary cases (i.e. no brain lesion seen on neuroimaging) labelled "TGA-p" [100] (see Sect. 2.2.3).

Many of the reports of brain tumour associated with TGA predate widely accepted clinical diagnostic criteria for TGA, and for this reason, some cases might be excluded as not conforming to the diagnosis. For example, in one case the amnesic episode lasted more than 24 h [84] and in another progressive memory problems

Table 7.4 Reports of concurrence of TGA with brain tumour (adapted from [16], p.106–8, and [40])

Reference	Patient details	Histology	Location
Aimard et al. (1971) [84]	F65	Glioblastoma	"Trigone and diffuse"
Hartley et al. (1974) [85]	M62	Chromophobe adenoma	Pituitary
Boudin et al. (1975) [86]	F73	Glioma	Posterior limbic system, bilateral
Lisak and Zimmerman (1977) [87]	M70	Unknown	L temporo-parietal
Shuping et al. (1980) [88]	M60	Glioblastoma	L hippocampus
Findler et al. (1983) [89]	M67	Metastasis	Non-dominant hemisphere
Meador et al. (1985) [90]	F47	Meningioma	R temporal lobe
Riva et al. (1985) [91]	F64	Meningioma	Olfactory bulb
Collins and Freeman (1986) [92]	M61	Meningioma	R parietal region
Matias-Guiu et al. (1986) [93]	M-	Unknown	R temporal lobe
Araga et al. (1989) [94]	F59	Meningioma	Falco-tentorial region
Cattaino et al. (1989) [95]	F47	Meningioma	R frontal lobe, ethmoidal
Po and Hseuh (1990) [96]	F65	Meningioma	R sphenoid ridge
Sorenson et al. (1995) [97]	F58	Astrocytoma	R hypothalamus
Honma and Nagao (1996) [98]	F68	Adenoma	Pituitary, complicated by haemorrhage
Huang and Pai (2008) [99]	M67	Unknown	L medial temporal lobe
Agosti et al. (2008) $n = 2$ [100]	–	Meningioma	Falx
Dinca et al. (2011) [101]	F75	Meningioma	R transtentorial (cerebellum to temporal lobe)
Na et al. (2019) [102]	M65	Adenoma	Pituitary, extending to L medial temporal lobe
Turki et al. (2020) [103]	F55	Unknown	R frontal lobe

followed a generalised tonic–clonic seizure [88]. One patient was reported to have six episodes of TGA and on examination had bilateral papilloedema [93]; this case was criticised as unlikely to be TGA by Hodges ([4], p.30). Caplan [104] had previously criticised the case reported by Meador et al. on the grounds that the reported clinical features (two short-lasting and unobserved episodes of loss of awareness) [90] did not suggest TGA, and Daniel thought the cases of Hartley et al. [85], Shuping et al. [88] and Honma and Nagao [98], associated respectively with a pituitary tumour, left temporal glioblastoma and chronic haematoma in a parasellar tumour compressing the right medial temporal lobe, were more likely to be transient epileptic amnesia (TEA; see Sect. 3.2), the first and last based on repeated episodes of amnesia ([105], p.187,188). This may also be the case with the patient reported by Huang and Pai [99] (Sect. 3.2.2).

Not all published descriptions of TGA and tumour can be admitted as such. For example, Ross reported a female patient (Case 3) aged about 65 years as "experiencing transient global amnesia". She had papilloedema and a right superior homonymous quadrantanopia and was eventually found to have a left temporal glioblastoma. However, the attacks of "unusual behaviour" labelled as TGA occurred 2–3 times per week, lasted 12–15 hours, had been experienced for about a year and were characterised by knowing no one, including herself [106]. These clinical features fall outwith current understanding of TGA, in terms of both the frequency and duration of episodes, and the loss of knowledge of self, not to mention the absence of any report of repetitive questioning, and accordingly, this case is not included, although other authors seem to have accepted it as a case of tumour-related TGA ([107], p.184).

In many of the reviewed cases, the finding of a tumour was deemed unlikely to be anything more than chance concurrence with TGA, based on tumour locations distant from memory-eloquent structures, and hence an entirely incidental finding [40]. A similar argument may be made with respect to other structural lesions identified in TGA patients, such as hydrocephalus [108, 109] or cyst [110], subdural haematomas [111] and cerebral angioma [112]. Hence to label these cases as "symptomatic TGA" would, in this author's view, be an error. Brain haematoma may on rare occasion (e.g. [113]) be relevant to an episode of TGA (Table 3.5).

For tumour locations more obviously of possible pathophysiological relevance, such as those involving medial temporal lobe structures (e.g. a pituitary adenoma extending to left medial temporal lobe and anterior hippocampus [102]), neoplastic lesions might be anticipated to result in abnormal electrical activity within these networks. Milburn-McNulty and Larner argued that localised tumours might lower the threshold for epileptiform events, which might masquerade clinically as TGA [40] (see also Case Study 7.2). In other words, they considered that "tumour-associated TGA" was in most, if not all, instances transient epileptic amnesia and not TGA (of note, the index case which prompted their systematic review [40] subsequently underwent diagnostic revision after long-term follow-up showed neuroradiological remission of the swelling in the amygdala region which had initially been thought to be a low-grade glioma [114]). In this context, it is of note that patients harbouring medial temporal lobe tumours [99, 115, 116] and amygdala swelling [117] have been described as manifesting episodes typical of both TGA and subsequently TEA.

Case Study 7.2: Brain Tumour and TGA?
The 79-year-old man reported in Case Study 2.1, who suffered a brief (ca. 30 minutes) amnesic episode whilst hiking which was suspected to be TGA but with no reliable witness account, hence failing to fulfil diagnostic criteria, was further assessed. On the Mini-Mental State Examination, he scored 26/30 and on the Six-item Cognitive Impairment Test (negatively scored) 10/28, dropping points for delayed recall on both these screening instruments. MR brain imaging showed a left temporal lobe mass lesion with surrounding vasogenic oedema, appearances consistent with a high-grade glioma. A possible epileptic aetiology for his transient amnesic episode now seemed more likely than TGA.

An account of five cases of TGA occurring several years after temporal lobec-tomy for epilepsy (related to hippocampal sclerosis or dysembryoplastic neuroepi-thelial tumour, DNET) has appeared, the episodes conforming to TGA diagnostic criteria [118]. Though designated by the authors as a precipitating factor, the signifi-cant delay between surgery and TGA would be more in keeping with a predisposing factor. Moreover, although these patients had been seizure-free after surgery, the possibility that these episodes were epileptic in origin, despite conforming to TGA diagnostic criteria, cannot be entirely discounted.

In addition to these structural lesions evident on clinical and/or neuroradiologi-cal grounds, it is also possible that microstructural changes within brain tissue and reorganised network hubs (e.g. [119]), as detected using sophisticated neuroimag-ing modalities such as voxel-based morphometry and diffusion tensor imaging (Sect. 5.1.3), may also increase vulnerability to, and hence constitute predisposing factors for, TGA.

7.13 Summary and Recommendations

Many possible predisposing factors for TGA have been examined. Of these, the most consistent observation seems to be a personal history of migraine but no factor has been shown to be necessary and/or sufficient to induce TGA. A greater under-standing of the neurobiology and hence the pathogenesis of TGA (see Chap. 9) might enlighten this field of research. Meantime, a number of more proximate, pre-cipitating factors for TGA, have been described and these are examined in the next chapter.

References

1. Hodges JR, Warlow CP. Syndromes of transient amnesia: towards a classification. A study of 153 cases. J Neurol Neurosurg Psychiatry. 1990;53:834–43.
2. Miller JW, Petersen RC, Metter EJ, Millikan CH, Yanagihara T. Transient global amnesia: clinical characteristics and prognosis. Neurology. 1987;37:733–7.
3. Koski KJ, Marttila RJ. Transient global amnesia: incidence in an urban population. Acta Neurol Scand. 1990;81:358–60.
4. Hodges JR. Transient amnesia. Clinical and neuropsychological aspects. London: WB Saunders; 1991.
5. Matias-Guiu J, Blanquer J, Falip R, Oltra A, Martin M. Incidence of transient global amnesia in Alcoi (Spain). Acta Neurol Scand. 1992;86:221.
6. Lauria G, Gentile M, Fassetta G, Casetta I, Caneve G. Incidence of transient global amnesia in the Belluno province, Italy: 1985 through 1995. Results of a community-based study. Acta Neurol Scand. 1997(95):303–10.
7. Berli R, Hutter A, Waespe W, Bachli EB. Transient global amnesia—not so rare after all. Swiss Med Wkly. 2009;139:288–92.

8. Brigo F, Lochner P, Tezzon F, Nardone R. Incidence of transient global amnesia in Merano, province of Bolzano. Italy Acta Neurol Belg. 2014;114:293–6.
9. Erba L, Czaplinski A. Transient global amnesia: an altitude sickness? Eur J Neurol. 2017;24(Suppl1):146. (EP1050)
10. Govoni V, Cesnik E, Ferri C, Fallica E. The distribution of the transient global amnesia in the province of Ferrara, Italy, a clue to the pathogenesis? Neurol Sci. 2021;42:1821–6.
11. Quinette P, Guillery-Girard B, Dayan J, de la Sayette V, Marquis S, Viader F, Desgranges B, Eustache F. What does transient global amnesia really mean? Review of the literature and thorough study of 142 cases. Brain. 2006;129:1640–58.
12. Keret O, Lev N, Steiner I. Seasonal changes in the incidence of transient global amnesia. Eur J Neurol. 2015;22(Suppl1):182. (abstract P1221)
13. Keret O, Lev N, Shochat T, Steiner I. Seasonal changes in the incidence of transient global amnesia. J Clin Neurol. 2016;12:403–6.
14. Hoyer C, Higashida K, Fabbian F, et al. Chronobiology of transient global amnesia. J Neurol. 2022;269:361–7.
15. Larner AJ. Seasonal incidence of transient global amnesia. Poster presentation, BNA/ABN Meeting of Minds symposium, Cardiff, UK, 29 September 2016.
16. Larner AJ. Transient global amnesia. From patient encounter to clinical neuroscience. London: Springer; 2017.
17. Akkawi NM, Agosti C, Grassi M, et al. Weather conditions and transient global amnesia. A six-year study. J Neurol. 2006;253:194–8.
18. Oehler E, Iaxx F, Larre P, Ghawche F. Transient global amnesia: a descriptive study of 12 Polynesian patients [in French]. Rev Neurol (Paris). 2015;171:662–8.
19. Garcia-Carrasco M, Galarza C, Gomez-Ponce M, et al. Antiphospholipid syndrome in Latin American patients: clinical and immunologic characteristics and comparison with European patients. Lupus. 2007;16:366–73.
20. Agosti C, Borroni B, Akkawi N, Padovani A. Cerebrovascular risk factors and triggers in transient global amnesia patients with and without jugular valve incompetence: results from a sample of 243 patients. Eur Neurol. 2010;63:291–4.
21. Ahn S, Kim W, Lee YS, et al. Transient global amnesia. seven years of experience with diffusion-weighted imaging in an emergency department. Eur Neurol. 2011;65:123–8.
22. Ryoo I, Kim JH, Kim S, Choi BS, Jung C, Hwang SI. Lesion detectability on diffusion-weighted imaging in transient global amnesia: the influence of imaging timing and magnetic field strength. Neuroradiology. 2012;54:329–34.
23. Döhring J, Schmuck A, Bartsch T. Stress-related factors in the emergence of transient global amnesia with hippocampal lesions. Front Behav Neurosci. 2014;8:287.
24. Arena JE, Brown RD, Mandrekar J, Rabinstein AA. Long-term outcome in patients with transient global amnesia: a population-based study. Mayo Clin Proc. 2017;92:399–405.
25. Alessandro L, Calandri IL, Fernandez Suarez M, et al. Transient global amnesia: clinical features and prognostic factors suggesting recurrence. Arq Neuropsiquiatr. 2019;77:3–9.
26. Higashida K, Okazaki S, Todo K, et al. A multicenter study of transient global amnesia for the better detection of magnetic resonance imaging abnormalities. Eur J Neurol. 2020;27:2117–24.
27. Morris KA, Rabinstein AA, Young NP. Factors associated with risk of recurrent transient global amnesia. JAMA Neurol. 2020;77:1551–8.
28. Szabo K, Hoyer C, Caplan LR, et al. Diffusion-weighted MRI in transient global amnesia and its diagnostic implications. Neurology. 2020;95:e206–12.
29. Zeman AZJ, Boniface SJ, Hodges JR. Transient epileptic amnesia: a description of the clinical and neuropsychological features in 10 cases and a review of the literature. J Neurol Neurosurg Psychiatry. 1998;64:435–43.
30. Amit R, Shapira Y, Flusser H, Aker M. Basilar migraine manifesting as transient global amnesia in a 9-year-old child. Headache. 1986;26:17–8.

31. Dinsmore WW, Callender ME. Juvenile transient global amnesia. J Neurol Neurosurg Psychiatry. 1983;46:876–7.
32. Gravlee JR, Barrett JJ. Transient global amnesia in a collegiate baseball player with type I diabetes mellitus: a case report. J Athl Train. 2011;46:319–21.
33. Jensen T. Transient global amnesia in childhood. Dev Med Child Neurol. 1980;22:654–8.
34. Tirman PJ, Woody RC. Transient global amnesia precipitated by emotion in an adolescent. J Child Neurol. 1988;3:185–8.
35. Tosi L, Righetti CA. Transient global amnesia and migraine in young people. Clin Neurol Neurosurg. 1997;99:63–5.
36. Larner AJ. Acute confusional migraine and transient global amnesia: variants of cognitive migraine? Int J Clin Pract. 2013;67:1066.
37. Larner AJ. Transient global amnesia in the district general hospital. Int J Clin Pract. 2007;61:255–8.
38. Lim R, Larner AJ. Transient global amnesia: is female sex a risk factor for hospitalisation? Eur J Neurol. 2008;15(suppl3):303. (abstract P2369)
39. Larner AJ. Amnesia as a sex-related adverse event. Br J Hosp Med. 2011;72:292–3.
40. Milburn-McNulty P, Larner AJ. Transient global amnesia and brain tumour: chance concurrence or aetiological association? Case report and systematic literature review. Case Rep Neurol. 2015;7:18–25.
41. Yi M, Sherzai AZ, Ani C, Shavlik D, Ghamsary M, Lazar E, Sherzai D. Strong association between migraine and transient global amnesia: a national inpatient sample analysis. J Neuropsychiatry Clin Neurosci. 2019;31:43–8.
42. Corston RN, Godwin-Austen RB. Transient global amnesia in four brothers. J Neurol Neurosurg Psychiatry. 1982;45:375–7.
43. Munro JM, Loizou LA. Transient global amnesia—familial incidence. J Neurol Neurosurg Psychiatry. 1982;45:1070.
44. Stracciari A, Rebucci GG. Transient global amnesia and migraine: familial incidence. J Neurol Neurosurg Psychiatry. 1986;49:716.
45. Dupuis MM, Pierre PH, Gonsette RE. Transient global amnesia and migraine in twin sisters. J Neurol Neurosurg Psychiatry. 1987;50:816–7.
46. Agosti C, Borroni B, Akkawi N, Padovani A. Three sisters covering the transient global amnesia spectrum. Int Psychogeriatr. 2007;19:987–9.
47. Vyhnalek M, Bojar M, Jerabek J, Hort J. Long lasting recurrent familiar [sic] transient global amnesia after betablocker withdrawal: case report. Neuro Endocrinol Lett. 2008;29:44–6.
48. Segers-van Rijn J, de Bruijn SFTM. Transient global amnesia: a genetic disorder? Eur Neurol. 2010;63:186–7.
49. Galovic M, Schilg L, Felbecker A. Familial clustering of transient global amnesia. Eur J Neurol. 2011;18(Suppl2):427. (abstract P2223)
50. Goossens C, Dupuis MJM, Evrard FL, Picard G, Jacquerye P, Ghysens O. Transient global amnesia and migraine in two sisters. J Neurol. 2011;258(Suppl1):S240. (abstract P847)
51. Maggioni F, Mainardi F, Bellamio M, Zanchin G. Transient global amnesia triggered by migraine in monozygotic twins. Headache. 2011;51:1305–8.
52. Davies RR, Larner AJ. Familial transient global amnesia. Case Rep Neurol. 2012;4:236–9.
53. Dupuis MM, Evrard F, de Bruijn S, et al. Is transient global amnesia (TGA) hereditary? J Neurol Sci. 2013;333(Suppl1):e664.
54. Dandapat S, Bhargava P, Ala TA. Familial transient global amnesia. Mayo Clin Proc. 2015;90:696–7.
55. Dupuis M, Vandeponseele M, Jacquerye P, et al. Familial transient global amnesia: report of 10 families. J Neurol Sci. 2017;381(Suppl):381.
56. Larner AJ. Recurrent transient global amnesia: Is there a link to familial history? Prog Neurol Psychiatry. 2017;21(4):17–9.
57. Larner AJ. Recurrent TGA: link to family history? Prog Neurol Psychiatry. 2018;22(1):18.

58. Paccagnella E, Gosavi TD, Neligan A, Walker M. Transient epileptic amnesia: an unusual case report. Poster presentation, BNA/ABN Meeting of Minds symposium, Cardiff, UK, 29 September 2016.
59. Rojas-Marcos I, Fernandez A, Caballero JA, Suarez A, Blanco A. Familial transient epileptic amnesia. Report of three siblings. J Neurol. 2012;259(Suppl1):S178. (abstract P672)
60. Evans JH. Transient loss of memory, an organic mental syndrome. Brain. 1966;89:539–48.
61. Frank G. Amnestic episodes in migraine. A contribution to the differential diagnosis of transient global amnesia (ictus amnésique) [in German]. Schweiz Arch Neurol Neurochir Psychiatr. 1976;118:253–74.
62. Caplan L, Chedru F, Lhermitte F, Mayman C. Transient global amnesia and migraine. Neurology. 1981;31:1167–70.
63. Zorzon M, Antonutti L, Mase G, Biasutti E, Vitrani B, Cazzato G. Transient global amnesia and transient ischemic attack. Natural history, vascular risk factors, and associated conditions. Stroke. 1995;26:1536–42.
64. Schmidtke K, Ehmsen L. Transient global amnesia and migraine. A case control study. Eur Neurol. 1998,40.9–14.
65. Lin KH, Chen YT, Fuh JL, et al. Migraine is associated with a higher risk of transient global amnesia: a nationwide cohort study. Eur J Neurol. 2014;21:718–24.
66. Liampas I, Siouras AS, Siokas V, et al. Migraine in transient global amnesia: a meta-analysis of observational studies. J Neurol. 2021; https://doi.org/10.1007/s00415-020-10363-y. Online ahead of print.
67. Liampas I, Raptopoulou M, Mpourlios S, et al. Factors associated with recurrent transient global amnesia: systematic review and pathophysiological insights. Rev Neurosci. 2021;32:751–65.
68. Noël A, Quinette P, Guillery-Girard B, et al. Psychopathological factors, memory disorders and transient global amnesia. Br J Psychiatry. 2008;193:145–51.
69. Neri M, Andermarcher E, De Vreese LP, Rubichi S, Sacchet C, Cipolli C. Transient global amnesia: memory and metamemory. Aging (Milano). 1995;7:423–9.
70. Inzitari D, Pantoni L, Lamassa M, Pallanti S, Pracucci G, Marini P. Emotional arousal and phobia in transient global amnesia. Arch Neurol. 1997;54:866–73.
71. Pantoni L, Bertini E, Lamassa M, Pracucci G, Inzitari D. Clinical features, risk factors, and prognosis in transient global amnesia: a follow-up study. Eur J Neurol. 2005;12:350–6.
72. Fischer M, Dressen T, Jorg JR. Pathogenesis of transient global amnesia—a psychological clinical study leads to a new hypothesis. J Neurol. 2006;253(suppl2):II/71. (abstract P279)
73. Werner R, Keller M, Woehrle JC. Increased incidence of transient global amnesia during the Covid-19 crisis? Neurol Res Pract. 2020;2(1):26.
74. Chen ST, Tang LM, Hsu WC, Lee TH, Ro LS, Wu YR. Clinical features, vascular risk factors, and prognosis for transient global amnesia in Chinese patients. J Stroke Cerebrovasc Dis. 1999;8:295–9.
75. Santos S, Lopez del Val J, Tejero C, Iniguez C, Lalana JM, Morales F. Transient global amnesia: a review of 58 cases [in Spanish]. Rev Neurol. 2000;30:1113–7.
76. Piñol-Ripoll G, de la Puerta G-MI, Martinez L, et al. A study of the risk factors in transient global amnesia and its differentiation from a transient ischemic attack [in Spanish]. Rev Neurol. 2005;41:513–6.
77. Romero JR, Mercado M, Beiser AS, et al. Transient global amnesia and neurological events: the Framingham Heart Study. Front Neurol. 2013;4:47.
78. Jang JW, Park SY, Hong JH, Park YH, Kim JE, Kim S. Different risk factor profiles between transient global amnesia and transient ischemic attack: a large case-control study. Eur Neurol. 2014;71:19–24.
79. Tuduri I, Carneado J, Fragoso M, Ortiz P, Jimenez-Ortiz C. Transient global amnesia and vascular risk factors [in Spanish]. Rev Neurol. 2000;30:418–21.

80. Toledo M, Pujadas F, Purroy F, Lara N, Quintana M, Alvarez-Sabin J. Recurrent transient global amnesia, a manifestation of ischemic cerebrovascular disease [in Spanish]. Med Clin (Barc). 2005;125:361–5. [Erratum Med Clin (Barc). 2006;126:316]
81. Toledo M, Pujadas F, Grivé E, Alvarez-Sabin J, Quintana M, Rovira A. Lack of evidence for arterial ischemia in transient global amnesia. Stroke. 2008;39:476–9.
82. Liampas I, Raptopoulou M, Siokas V, et al. Conventional cardiovascular risk factors in transient global amnesia: systematic review and proposition of a novel hypothesis. Front Neuroendocrinol. 2021;61:100909.
83. Rogalewski A, Beyer A, Friedrich A, et al. Transient global amnesia (TGA): influence of acute hypertension in patients not adapted to chronic hypertension. Front Neurol. 2021;12:666632.
84. Aimard G, Trillet M, Perroudou C, Tommasi M, Carrier H. Ictus amnesique symptomatique d'un glioblastome interessant le trigone. Rev Neurol. 1971;124:392–6.
85. Hartley TC, Heilman KM, Garcia-Bengochea F. A case of transient global amnesia due to a pituitary tumor. Neurology. 1974;24:998–1000.
86. Boudin G, Pepin B, Mikol J, Haguenau M, Vernant JC. Gliome du systeme limbique posterieur, revele par une amnesia globale transitoire. Observation anatomo-clinique d'un cas. Rev Neurol. 1975;131:157–63.
87. Lisak RP, Zimmerman RA. Transient global amnesia due to a dominant hemisphere tumor. Arch Neurol. 1977;34:317–8.
88. Shuping JR, Toole JF, Alexander E Jr. Transient global amnesia due to a glioma in the dominant hemisphere. Neurology. 1980;30:88–90.
89. Findler G, Feinsod M, Lijovetzky G, Hadani M. Transient global amnesia associated with a single metastasis in the non-dominant hemisphere. Case report. J Neurosurg. 1983;58:303–5.
90. Meador KM, Adams RJ, Flanigin HF. Transient global amnesia and meningioma. Neurology. 1985;35:769–71.
91. Riva C, Leiva C, Gobernado JM, Gimeno A. Amnesia global transitoria asociada a un meningioma del lobulo frontal. Med Clin (Barc). 1985;84:81.
92. Collins MP, Freeman JW. Meningioma and transient global amnesia: another report. Neurology. 1986;36:594.
93. Matias-Guiu J, Colomer R, Segura A, Codina A. Cranial CT scan in transient global amnesia. Acta Neurol Scand. 1986;73:298–301.
94. Araga S, Fukada M, Kagimoto H, Imagawa T, Takahashi K. Transient global amnesia and falcotentorial meningioma—a case report. Jpn J Psychiatry Neurol. 1989;43:201–3.
95. Cattaino G, Pomes A, Querin F, Cecotto C. Ethmoidal meningioma revealed by transient global amnesia. Ital J Neurol Sci. 1989;10:187–91.
96. Po HL, Hseuh IH. Transient global amnesia associated with a right sphenoid ridge meningioma: a case report. Zhonghua Yi Xue Za Zhi (Taipei). 1990;46:113–6.
97. Sorenson EJ, Silbert PL, Benarroch EE, Jack CR, Parisi JE. Transient amnesic syndrome after spontaneous haemorrhage into a hypothalamic pilocytic astrocytoma. J Neurol Neurosurg Psychiatry. 1995;58:761–3.
98. Honma Y, Nagao S. Hemorrhagic pituitary adenoma manifesting as transient global amnesia. Neurol Med Chir (Tokyo). 1996;36:234–6.
99. Huang CF, Pai MC. Transient amnesia in a patient with left temporal tumor. Symptomatic transient global amnesia or an epileptic amnesia? Neurologist. 2008;14:196–200.
100. Agosti C, Borroni B, Akkawi NM, De Maria G, Padovani A. Transient global amnesia and brain lesions: new hints into clinical criteria. Eur J Neurol. 2008;15:981–4.
101. Dinca EB, Carron R, Gay E. Transient global amnesia as a revealing sign of giant transtentorial meningioma. Case report and review of the literature. J Nerv Ment Dis. 2011;199:416–8.
102. Na S, Lee ES, Lee SJ. Transient global amnesia in a patient with pituitary adenoma: causal or chance association? Case Rep Neurol. 2019;11:238–41.
103. Turki BG, Ozdemir AF, Isler C. A rare case of transient global amnesia caused by a brain tumor. Eur J Neurol. 2020;27(Suppl1):1066. (abstract EPO3081)
104. Caplan LR. Transient global amnesia: criteria and classification. Neurology. 1986;36:441.

105. Daniel BT. Transient global amnesia. Print version and ebook: Amazon; 2012.
106. Ross RT. Transient tumor attacks. Arch Neurol. 1983;40:633–6.
107. Simos PG, Papanicolaou AC. Transient global amnesia. In: Papanicolaou AC, editor. The amnesias: a clinical textbook of memory disorders. Oxford: Oxford University Press; 2006. p. 171–89.
108. Giroud M, Guard O, Dumas R. Transient global amnesia associated with hydrocephalus. Report of two cases. J Neurol. 1987;235:118–9.
109. Rocha S, Pinho J, Rito M, Machado A. Expanding Virchow-Robin spaces; transient global amnesia and obstructive hydrocephalus. J Neuropsychiatry Clin Neurosci. 2013;25:E49–50.
110. Stracciari A, Ciucci G, Bissi G. Transient global amnesia associated with a large arachnoid cyst of the middle cranial fossa of the non dominant hemisphere. Ital J Neurol Sci. 1987;8:609–11.
111. Chatham PE, Brillman J. Transient global amnesia associated with bilateral subdural hematomas. Neurosurgery. 1985;17:971–3.
112. Heine P, Degos JD, Meyrignac C. Cerebral angioma disclosed by 2 episodes of transient global amnesia [in French]. Presse Med. 1986;15:1049.
113. Moonis M, Jain S, Prasad K, Mishra NK, Goulatia RK, Maheshwari MC. Left thalamic hypertensive haemorrhage presenting as transient global amnesia. Acta Neurol Scand. 1988;77:331–4.
114. Larner AJ. Transient epileptic amnesia and amygdala enlargement revisited. Psychogeriatrics. 2021;21:943–4.
115. Fouchard AA, Biberon J, Mondon K, de Toffol B. Transient epileptic amnesia secondary to hippocampal dysplasia mimicking transient global amnesia. Seizure. 2016;43:23–5.
116. Sugiyama A, Kobayashi M, Matsunaga T, Kanai T, Kuwabara S. Transient global amnesia with a hippocampal lesion followed by transient epileptic amnesia. Seizure. 2015;31:141–3.
117. Kanbayahsi T, Hatanaka Y, Sonoo M. Transient epileptic amnesia with amygdala enlargement. Neurol Sci. 2020;41:1591–3.
118. Dupont S, Samson S, Baulac M. Is anterior temporal lobectomy a precipitating factor for transient global amnesia? J Neurol Neurosurg Psychiatry. 2008;79:309–11.
119. Park KM, Lee BI, Kim SE. Is transient global amnesia a network disease? Eur Neurol. 2018;80:345–54.

Chapter 8
Epidemiology of TGA (2): Possible Precipitating Factors

Abstract This chapter examines factors identified in clinical and epidemiological studies as possible precipitating factors for episodes of TGA. Of these, emotional stress and physical effort are the most commonly identified. It is possible that these precipitating factors may give some insights into the pathogenesis of TGA. Predisposing factors for TGA are considered in the previous chapter.

Keywords TGA · Precipitating factors

A number of factors have been described in close temporal association with (i.e. immediately before) the onset of an attack of TGA and hence may be designated as precipitating factors, as opposed to those with a more distant temporal association which may be designated predisposing factors (Chap. 7). Miller Fisher identified such precipitating factors in 26/85 TGA episodes (30.6%) [1], whilst Rösler et al. identified precipitants in 58% of their 72 TGA patients based on administration of a standardised questionnaire [2]. In their review of cases reported in the literature, Quinette et al. noted precipitating factors in 462 of 881 cases (= 52.4%) and in their own series in 131 of 147 episodes (= 89.1%) [3]. Cejas et al. identified triggering factors in 41/79 (51.9%) of their TGA patients who agreed to complete a questionnaire [4], and in a retrospective survey of 389 patients, Hoyer et al. identified a precipitating factor in 266 (68.4%) [5]. Morris et al. found a similar percentage of cases with identifiable triggers in single-episode (28.8%) and recurrent (35.0%) TGA [6].

8.1 Emotional Stress

In his report on a series of 85 episodes of TGA, Miller Fisher found that highly emotional experiences were found to be the most common recognised precipitating event (8/26) [1]. Hodges and Warlow noted an emotionally stressful event in the 24 h before an episode of TGA in 14% of their prospective sample, examples including receiving bad news, witnessing an accident or being involved in an argument

[7]. Emotional arousal was also noted as a precipitating factor for TGA by Merriam and colleagues [8, 9] who emphasised the differentiation of TGA from the forms of transient psychological amnesia (Sect. 3.3) which may also follow stressful experiences. Quinette et al. noted that emotionally charged events may be a precipitant of TGA, reported in 28% of cases in their literature survey and in 29% of their personally observed cases [3]. Emotional stress may be a predisposing factor for as well as precipitating event to TGA (Sect. 7.10).

The specific emotional stress may take many various forms, including the experience of a burglary [10], a disturbing dream [11] or an emotionally charged psychotherapy session [12]. A similar explanation might account for TGA following general anaesthesia in an anxious patient undergoing otolaryngological surgery [13].

Quinette et al. reported that TGA in women was mainly associated with an emotional precipitating event (cf. men, physical precipitating event) [3]. In a retrospective study of a cohort of 389 TGA patients, Hoyer et al. examined gender-related differences in stressful precipitating events and confirmed that emotional triggers were more often experienced by women (37.2% vs. 22.8%) [5]. Noh and Kang reported "extreme stress" occurring in 64.6% of their cohort of TGA patients, most of whom (114/128 = 89%) were women [14].

8.2   Physical Effort

Many forms of physical exercise have been described as precipitating factors for TGA, including cycling (e.g. [15, 16]; see also Case Studies 2.1 and 7.1), swimming (e.g. [17], and [18], case 2), skiing ([19]; also Case Study 7.1), gardening/digging (e.g. [4, 20]), sawing wood, after extreme exercise (e.g. [21]) and after medical procedures involving an exercise testing procedure such as the bicycle ergometer or treadmill [22, 23]. Other recorded effortful activities include defecation in constipated patients, coughing, vomiting and repeated yawning [4].

Hodges reported exercise as a precipitant in 18% of patients in the Oxford TGA study ([24], p.19). Quinette et al. noted physical effort as a precipitant of TGA in 31% of cases in their literature survey and in 25% of their personally observed cases [3]. Hoyer et al. found physical stressors were more common in men than women (41.1% vs. 30.7%) [5]. Hence, physical triggers of TGA are more often experienced by men and emotional triggers more often by women.

8.3   Water Contact or Temperature Change

Fisher and Adams "first case" (see Sect. 1.1) was associated with a swim in cold water [25]. In a report on a series of 85 episodes of TGA, Fisher found that bathing in cold water (specifically the Atlantic Ocean) was found to be a common recognised precipitating event (3/26) [1]. Other examples have also been reported (e.g. Case Studies 2.1 and 6.1). Quinette et al. reported water contact or temperature change (which could include hot baths) in 14% of patients in their literature review and in 11% of their own series [3]. Martin coined the term "amnesia by the seaside" for TGA cases associated with cold water immersion [26]. Tubridy et al. also used the term [27], even when there was no cold water immersion, merely a walk by the seaside ([28], p.11–6).

An episode of transient amnesia in a volunteer undergoing experimental repeated cold water (20 °C) immersion has been reported as TGA [29], but the details are not convincing for this diagnosis, specifically the development of "altered affect … whimpering, anxious delirium-like state" for 20 min. It was also atypical in the subject's age (23).

Temperature change might also possibly contribute to or explain TGA cases associated with skiing ([19]; Case Study 7.1), high altitude [30–32], transoceanic flight [33], paragliding [34], infusion of cryopreserved cells [35] and whole-body cryotherapy (brief exposure to very cold and dry air) [36]. A study from relatively high altitude (Davos, Switzerland) found TGA cases peaked in the winter, suggesting that low temperature might be either a predisposing factor or a trigger for TGA, but no relation was found with atmospheric pressure, wind or humidity [37].

8.4 Sexual Activity

Amnesia is one of the recognised acute neurological consequences of sexual activity, as is headache, but whether these are separate or pathophysiologically related conditions is not currently known [38].

Sexual activity was noted as a precipitating factor for TGA in 2/17 patients reported by Fisher and Adams [25], and in a later report on a series of 85 episodes of TGA, Fisher found it to be the second most common recognised precipitating event for TGA (7/26) [1]. Hodges and Warlow reported sexual intercourse to be the precipitant of TGA in 3% of their cases [7]. Quinette et al. reported sexual intercourse as a precipitant in 12% of patients in their literature review and in 9% of their own series [3].

In addition, many individual possible reports of "coital" or "post-coital" amnesia have also been presented (e.g. [39–51].; see also Case Study 4.1 and Case Study 8.1). These include examples of recurrent episodes of amnesia after intercourse [52–54].

Case Study 8.1: Sexual Activity as a Precipitating Factor of TGA
A previously healthy 61-year-old man had an episode of memory loss. Somewhat abashed, he reported that about 7 weeks earlier he and his wife had been making love at 5 o'clock in the morning, "not something we usually do". He then got up and was found in the kitchen some minutes later by his wife. She reported that he was repeatedly asking "where am I?". Questioned by her, he had forgotten the names of his medications for high blood pressure and the fact that his son had recently passed his driving test. However, these functions returned after a period of about 4 h and did not recur. His general practitioner made a provisional diagnosis of transient ischaemic attack (TIA). The patient was commenced on aspirin, non-urgent structural brain imaging was arranged and referral made to the neurology clinic (adapted from [45]).

Monzani et al. reported on 10 patients (all male; age range 41–64 years) with transient amnesia related to sexual activity, which comprised 18% of all acute global amnesia patients observed during the study period; of these ten, one had a subarachnoid haemorrhage whilst all the others were diagnosed as TGA [55].

Episodes of TGA reported in association with the use of phosphodiesterase type 5 (PDE-5) inhibitors, sildenafil (Viagra) and tadalafil, and with the intracavernosal injection of alprostadil (Caverject) (Sect. 3.4.2 and Table 3.8), may also be precipitated by sexual activity rather than being an acute adverse drug effect.

Concurrence of sex-related TGA and primary headache associated with sexual activity (PHSA), whose features differ from migraine, has been reported on occasion [56–58]. This may suggest the possibility either of shared pathophysiological mechanisms, perhaps related to activation of pathways within the trigeminocervical complex [58] or a concurrence of two disorders with a shared trigger [57].

8.5   Pain

In a report on a series of 85 episodes of TGA, pain was found to be one of the most common recognised precipitating events (6/26) [1]. Examples may include abdominal pain [25], dental extraction [59], trigeminal ganglion stimulation ([1], in 2/26), pain from a pilonidal sinus ([24], p.18) and myocardial infarction, although TGA after painless MI has also been reported (Sect. 3.1.6). TGA associated with other painful medical procedures is also well described (Sect. 8.8). Quinette et al. noted acute pain as a precipitant of TGA in 2% of cases in their literature survey and in 3% of their personally observed cases [3].

Migraine headache is a not infrequent accompaniment of TGA episodes, possibly as a precipitant (Sect. 8.6), as well as being a predisposing factor (Sect. 7.9) and a symptomatic cause of amnesia which enters the differential diagnosis of TGA (Sect. 3.4.1). Whether the pain associated with migraine headache per se may be considered a precipitant of TGA, rather than the migraine pathophysiology, does not seem to be commented upon in the literature.

The absence of case reports of TGA related to events acknowledged to be associated with severe pain such as parturition or cluster headache might be taken to argue against pain per se as a precipitant. Nephrolithiasis or ureteral colic is a rarely reported association with TGA [1, 60]. Fisher and Adams ([25], p.40) reported "One woman was in the throes of rather severe ureteral colic (this patient thought two of her previous attacks had also been precipitated by pain)". Another possible association of TGA and kidney stone was confounded by use of multiple doses of opioid and non-opioid analgesia [61].

8.6   Migraine

Migraine has already been discussed in the context of the differential diagnosis of TGA (Sect. 3.4.1) and as a possible predisposing factor for TGA (Sect. 7.9). It may also be a precipitating factor.

TGA occurring during a migraine attack has been reported by many authors (e.g. [62–68]. However, this is probably a very rare occurrence. A large retrospective analysis from a centre in France identified six cases of TGA occurring (hence, according to the paper's title, "triggered") by a migraine attack amongst a cohort of 8821 new patients seen over an 11-year period [69]. Other mechanisms might also be envisaged, for example forceful vomiting in the context of a migraine attack might be associated with the Valsalva manoeuvre (Sect. 8.9).

Many of the familial examples of TGA (Sect. 7.8) had TGA episodes which reportedly occurred at the same time as a migraine (see Table 7.3).

8.7 Brain Infections

Brain infections are included amongst the symptomatic causes of amnesia (Sect. 3.5.2; Table 3.2) and may enter the differential diagnosis of TGA. Cases labelled diagnostically as "TGA" have on occasion been reported in association with infective disorders of the brain, including herpes simplex encephalitis [70, 71], neurosyphilis [72] and Epstein–Barr virus encephalitis [73], although Daniel states that these latter authors "clearly described a case of transient epileptic amnesia" ([74], p.205).

8.8 Medical Procedures and Therapies

Onset of TGA concurrent with the performance of various medical procedures has been described. Of these, angiography (cerebral, coronary) appears to be the most frequently described (see Sect. 3.1.5; Table 3.6).

Angiography was recognised as a possible precipitating event for transient amnesia even before the TGA nomenclature was coined ([75]; see Sect. 1.2). A retrospective analysis of over 20,000 angiographic procedures undertaken at one hospital over a period of 7.5 years identified 9 cases of TGA (= 0.04%), which followed either cerebral angiography (5 in 4360 = 0.11%) or cardiac angiography (4 in 8817 = 0.05%) but no cases following peripheral angiography were identified (0 in 7659), indicating the infrequency of the association of TGA with angiography [76]. Even cardiologists with extensive (>25 years) experience of cardiac angiography, encompassing many thousands of procedures, may not encounter a case of TGA (Dr WL Morrison, personal communication, Liverpool Heart and Chest Hospital, 24/12/16).

Various other medical procedures have sometimes been associated with the onset of TGA (Table 8.1). For example, upper gastrointestinal endoscopic procedures have on occasion been followed by TGA (e.g. [85, 87, 89, 90]), as has transoesophageal echocardiography [82, 83]. Possible explanations might include the emotional stress of instrumentation, associated pain, autonomic activation from passing the

Table 8.1 Reports of medical procedures associated with onset of TGA (see text for caveats)

Procedure	Reference(s)
Acupuncture	Hodges (1991) ($n = 1$) ([24], p.18)
Anaesthesia	Ghoneim (1998) [77]
	Bortolon et al. (2005) [78]
	Galipienzo et al. (2012) [13]
Aneurysm coiling	Graff-Radford et al. (2013) [79]
Angiography(cerebral, coronary)	See Table 3.6
Carotid artery stenting	Lee (2020) [80]
Cryotherapy	Carrard et al. (2017) [36]
Cystoscopy	Miller et al. (1987) [22]
Deep brain stimulation (misplaced electrode)	Baezner et al. (2013) [81]
Dental extraction	Godlewski (1968) [59]
Echocardiogram (transoesophageal)	Profice et al. (2008) [82]
	Cassar and Balkhausen (2020) [83]
Electroencephalography (EEG)	Cole et al. (1987) [84]
	Ung and Larner (2014) [50]
Endoscopy(upper gastrointestinal)	Hiraga and Matsunaga (2006) ($n = 3$) [85]
	Neuzillet et al. (2009) [86]
	Sayilir et al. (2009) [87]
	Ahn et al. (2011) ($n = 4$) [88]
	Cesar and Perdigao (2012) [89]
	Jeong et al. (2018) ($n = 2$) [90]
Exercise testing(cycle ergometer, treadmill)	Miller et al. (1987) [22]
	Richardson et al. (1998) [23]
Intracarotid amobarbital procedure	Benke et al. (2005) [91]
Nasogastric tube insertion	Miller et al. (1987) [22]
Nasopharyngeal swab	Ravaglia et al. (2021) [92]
"Oral provocation test" (rofecoxib)	Hirschfeld et al. (2007) [93]
Photodynamic therapy	Reinholz et al. (2015) [94]
Psychotherapy	Espiridion et al. (2019) [12]
Pulmonary function testing	Miller et al. (1987) [22]
	Robbins et al. (2010) [95]
	Williamson and Larner (2016) [96]
Radio frequency catheter ablation for premature cardiac ventricular beats	Mokabberi et al. (2010) [97]
Stellate ganglion block	Park et al. (2015) [98]
Stem cell infusion (autologous peripheral blood)	Otrock et al. (2008) [35]
Trigeminal ganglion stimulation	Fisher (1982) ($n = 2$) [1]
Urinary catheterisation	Ahn et al. (2011) ($n = 1$) [88]
Urography (excretory)	Miller et al. (1987) [22]
Venesection	Hodges (1991) ($n = 2$) ([24], p.18)

scope and medication use (scopolamine in [85], although TGA is also recorded following endoscopy without medication [87]). No account of TGA after colonoscopy has been identified.

A review by Jeong et al. published in 2018 found 89 patients with medical procedure-related TGA described in 49 articles. The most common procedure was angiography (cerebral > coronary) followed by general anaesthesia, although with only nine cases the latter could simply be chance. Neurological procedures were more common than cardiac, anaesthetic, gastrointestinal and pulmonary procedures. The authors concluded that Valsalva-associated activities, emotional stress with anxiety and acute pain were predisposing (sic) conditions in these cases [90]. Hoyer et al. recorded TGA following a medical procedure in 2.1% of their cohort of 389 patients [5].

All these accounts of TGA associated with medical procedures are rare, considering the frequency with which the various procedures are undertaken, so could be chance concurrence rather than causal association. Moreover, medical procedures are often accompanied by patient emotional stress (e.g. psychotherapy [12]), particularly anxiety (Sect. 8.1) and pain (Sect. 8.5), which might also be contributory factors in the cases observed.

8.9 Valsalva Manoeuvre

Bedside spirometry (forced vital capacity), one of the medical procedures reported on occasion to precipitate an episode of TGA [22, 95, 96] (Sect. 8.8), requires breath holding before forced expiration, effectively the performance of a Valsalva manoeuvre. This manoeuvre has sometimes been implicated in a number of other situations associated with TGA onset, including physical exercise, sexual activity, cold water immersion and response to pain. It has also been considered relevant to the retrograde internal jugular vein blood flow due to jugular vein valve incompetence (Sect. 4.3.3.2) which is pertinent to one of the hypotheses of TGA pathogenesis (Sect. 9.2.2).

However, attempts to reproduce the typical clinical and neuroradiological findings of TGA by voluntary Valsalva manoeuvre have failed. Patients with a previous episode of TGA were subjected to a controlled Valsalva manoeuvre, at least 3 months post-event, and suffered no recurrence of either typical symptoms or MR-DWI findings of TGA [99]. Jeong et al. noted that more than half of their patients ($n = 8$) with incidental MR-DWI hippocampal hyperintensities had performed Valsalva manoeuvre-associated activities but this was also true of their TGA group ($n = 16$) [100].

Valsalva manoeuvre may thus be an associated, rather a precipitating, factor in some episodes of TGA.

8.10   Other Possible Precipitating Factors

TGA cases associated with medication use have been reported on occasion (Table 3.8). These drugs might possibly be considered as precipitating factors, but the paucity of reports and the variety of drugs suggest no one specific class of drugs as being particularly culpable. Emerging pharmacovigilance data suggest COVID-19 vaccines may be an exception.

There have been occasional reports of TGA occurring at high altitude [30–32] suggesting a possible role for cerebral hypoxia, although physical effort and temperature change may be contributory (and/or confounding) factors in these cases.

8.11   Summary and Recommendations

Many possible precipitating factors for TGA have been examined. Some consistent observations have been made, but no factor seems to be necessary and/or sufficient to induce TGA. This has prompted various aetiological theories for TGA which are reviewed and elaborated upon in the next chapter.

References

1. Fisher CM. Transient global amnesia. Precipitating activities and other observations. Arch Neurol. 1982;39:605–8.
2. Rösler A, Mras GJ, Frese A, Albert I, Schnorpfeil F. Precipitating factors of transient global amnesia. J Neurol. 1999;246:53–4.
3. Quinette P, Guillery-Girard B, Dayan J, de la Sayette V, Marquis S, Viader F, Desgranges B, Eustache F. What does transient global amnesia really mean? Review of the literature and thorough study of 142 cases. Brain. 2006;129:1640–58.
4. Cejas C, Cisneros LF, Lagos R, Zuk C, Ameriso SF. Internal jugular vein valve incompetence is highly prevalent in transient global amnesia. Stroke. 2010;41:67–71.
5. Hoyer C, Ebert A, Sandicki V, Platten M, Szabo K. Sex-related differences in stressful events precipitating transient global amnesia—a retrospective observational study. J Neurol Sci. 2021;425:117464.
6. Morris KA, Rabinstein AA, Young NP. Factors associated with risk of recurrent transient global amnesia. JAMA Neurol. 2020;77:1551–8.
7. Hodges JR, Warlow CP. Syndromes of transient amnesia: towards a classification. A study of 153 cases. J Neurol Neurosurg Psychiatry. 1990;53:834–43.
8. Merriam AE. Emotional arousal-induced transient global amnesia. Case report, differentiation from hysterical amnesia, and an etiologic hypothesis. Neuropsychiatry Neuropsychol. Behav Neurol. 1988;1:73–8.
9. Merriam AE, Wyszynski B, Betzler T. Emotional arousal-induced transient global amnesia. A clue to the neural transcription of emotion? Psychosomatics. 1992;33:109–13.
10. Pillmann F, Broich K. Transitory global amnesia – psychogenic origin of organic disease? Psychopathologic basis and pathogenetic considerations [in German]. Fortschr Neurol Psychiatr. 1998;66:160–3.

11. Marinella MA. Transient global amnesia and a father's worst nightmare. N Engl J Med. 2004;350:843–4.
12. Espiridion ED, Gupta J, Bshara A, Danssaert Z. Transient global amnesia in a 60-year-old female with post-traumatic stress disorder. Cureus. 2019;11(9):e5792.
13. Galipienzo J, Lablanca MS, Zannin I, Rosado R, Zarza B, Olarra J. Transient global amnesia after general anaesthesia. Rev Esp Anestesiol Reanim. 2012;59:335–8.
14. Noh SM, Kang HG. Clinical manifestation and imaging characteristics of transient global amnesia: patent foramen ovale as an underlying factor. J Integr Neurosci. 2021;20:719–25.
15. Milburn-McNulty P, Larner AJ. Transient global amnesia and brain tumour: chance concurrence or aetiological association? Case report and systematic literature review. Case Rep Neurol. 2015;7:18–25.
16. Shuping JR, Rollinson RD, Toole JF. Transient global amnesia. Ann Neurol. 1980;7:281–5.
17. Jeong HS, Moon JS, Baek IC, Lee AY, Kim JM. Transient global amnesia with post-hyperventilation temporal sharp waves—a case report. Seizure. 2010;19:609–11.
18. Sakashita Y, Sugimoto T, Taki S, Matsuda H. Abnormal cerebral blood flow following transient global amnesia. J Neurol Neurosurg Psychiatry. 1993;56:1327.
19. Ay H, Furie KL, Yamada K, Koroshetz WJ. Diffusion-weighted MRI characterizes the ischemic lesion in transient global amnesia. Neurology. 1998;51:901–3.
20. Corston RN, Godwin-Austen RB. Transient global amnesia in four brothers. J Neurol Neurosurg Psychiatry. 1982;45:375–7.
21. Magazi D. Amnesia after a half marathon—a case study. Clin J Sport Med. 2012;22:448–9.
22. Miller JW, Petersen RC, Metter EJ, Millikan CH, Yanagihara T. Transient global amnesia: clinical characteristics and prognosis. Neurology. 1987;37:733–7.
23. Richardson RS, Leek BT, Wagner PD, Kritchevsky M. Transient global amnesia: a complication of incremental exercise testing. Med Sci Sports Exerc. 1998;30(10Suppl):S403-5.
24. Hodges JR. Transient amnesia. Clinical and neuropsychological aspects. London: WB Saunders; 1991.
25. Fisher CM, Adams RD. Transient global amnesia. Acta Neurol Scand. 1964;40(Suppl9):1–81.
26. Martin EA. Transient global amnesia. A report of eleven cases, including five of amnesia at the seaside. Ir J Med Sci. 1970;3:331–5.
27. Tubridy N, Hutchinson M, Murphy RP. Transient global amnesia: "amnesia by the seaside" revisited. J Neurol. 1999;246:500–1.
28. Tubridy N. Just one more question. Stories from a life in neurology. London: Penguin Ireland; 2019.
29. Castellani JW, Young AJ, Sawka MN, Backus VL, Canete JJ. Amnesia during cold water immersion: a case report. Wilderness Environ Med. 1998;9:153–5.
30. Bucuk M, Tomic Z, Tuskan-Mohar L, Bonifacic D, Bralic M, Jurjevic A. Recurrent transient global amnesia at high altitude. High Alt Med Biol. 2008;9:239–40.
31. Litch JA, Bishop RA. Transient global amnesia at high altitude. N Engl J Med. 1999;340:1444.
32. Litch JA, Bishop RA. High-altitude global amnesia. Wilderness Environ Med. 2000;11:25–8.
33. Rashid J, Starer PJ. Transient global amnesia following a transoceanic flight. Psychiatry Clin Neurosci. 2006;60:516–20.
34. Milheiro I, Rocha S, Machado A. Falling (or ascending) into oblivion: transient global amnesia with paragliding. J Neuropsychiatry Clin Neurosci. 2011;23:E40.
35. Otrock ZK, Beydoun A, Barada WM, Masroujeh R, Hourani R, Bazarbachi A. Transient global amnesia associated with the infusion of DMSO-cryopreserved autologous peripheral blood stem cells. Haematologica. 2008;93:e36–7.
36. Carrard J, Lambert AC, Genné D. Transient global amnesia following a whole-body crytotherapy session. BMJ Case Rep. 2018;2017:bcr2017221431.
37. Erba L, Czaplinski A. Transient global amnesia: an altitude sickness? Eur J Neurol. 2017;24(Suppl1):146 (EP1050)
38. Larner AJ. Transient acute neurologic sequelae of sexual activity: headache and amnesia. J Sex Med. 2008;5:284–8.

39. Agosti C, Borroni B, Akkawi N, Padovani A. Three sisters covering the transient global amnesia spectrum. Int Psychogeriatr. 2007;19:987–9.
40. Alonso-Navarro H, Jimenez-Jimenez FJ. Transient global amnesia during sexual intercourse [in Spanish]. Rev Neurol. 2006;42:382–3.
41. Bucuk M, Muzur A, Willheim K, Jurjevic A, Tomic Z, Tuskan ML. Make love to forget: two cases of transient global amnesia triggered by sexual intercourse. Coll Anthropol. 2004;28:899–905.
42. Dandapat S, Bhargava P, Ala TA. Familial transient global amnesia. Mayo Clin Proc. 2015;90:696–7.
43. Dang CV, Gardner LB. Transient global amnesia after sex. Lancet. 1998;352:1557–8.
44. Gallagher J, Murphy MS, Carroll J. Transient global amnesia after sexual intercourse. Ir J Med Sci. 2005;174:86–7.
45. Larner AJ. Amnesia as a sex-related adverse event. Br J Hosp Med. 2011;72:292–3.
46. Maloy K, Davis JE. "Forgettable" sex: a case of transient global amnesia presenting to the emergency department. J Emerg Med. 2011;41:257–60.
47. Marques-Vilallonga A, Aranda-Rodriguez S, Trallero-Araguas E, Jimenez-Moreno FX. Transient global amnesia associated to sildenafil and sexual activity [in Spanish]. Rev Neurol. 2014;59:93.
48. Mayeux R. Sexual intercourse and transient global amnesia. N Engl J Med. 1979;300:864.
49. Okura M, Nakayama H, Nagamine I, Ikuta T. Sexual intercourse as a precipitating factor of transient global amnesia. Jpn J Psychiatry Neurol. 1993;47:13–6.
50. Ung KYC, Larner AJ. Transient amnesia: epileptic or global? A differential diagnosis with significant implications for management. Q J Med. 2014;107:915–7.
51. Velasco R, Al-Hussayni S, Bermejo PE. Sexual intercourse as a trigger of transient global amnesia [in Spanish]. Rev Neurol. 2008;47:301–3.
52. Bermejo PE, García-Cobos E. Recurrent post-coital transient global amnesia. Rev Neurol. 2010;51:316–7.
53. Gonzalez-Martinez V, Comte F, de Verbizier D, Carlander B. Transient global amnesia: concordant hippocampal abnormalities on positron emission tomography and magnetic resonance imaging. Arch Neurol. 2010;67:510–1.
54. Lane RJ. Recurrent coital amnesia. J Neurol Neurosurg Psychiatry. 1997;63:260.
55. Monzani V, Rovellini A, Schinco G, Silani V. Transient global amnesia or subarachnoid haemorrhage? Clinical and laboratory findings in a particular type of acute global amnesia. Eur J Emerg Med. 2000;7:291–3.
56. Antunes F, Rosário Marques I, Grunho MD. Sex, headache and amnesia: filling in the blanks. Eur J Neurol. 2015;22(Suppl1):833. (abstract D168)
57. Knapen SE, Onderwater GL, Roon KI. Double whammy: a concurrence of two disorders with a shared trigger. Acta Neurol Belg. 2020;120:993–4.
58. Ziso B, Larner AJ. Double whammy: sex-related headache and amnesia. Acta Neurol Belg. 2020;120:699.
59. Godlewski S. Amnesic episodes (transient global amnesia). (clinical study based on 33 unpublished cases) [in French]. Sem Hop. 1968;44:553–77.
60. Kettaneh A, Gobron C, Fain O, Mohib S, Thomas M. Calculi and memory. Eur J Neurol. 2001;8:195–6.
61. Durrani M, Milas J, Parson G, Pescatore R. Temporary memory steal: transient global amnesia secondary to nephrolithiasis. Clin Pract Cases Emerg Med. 2018;2:334–7.
62. Caffarra P, Scaglioni A, Malvezzi L, Manzoni GM. Transient global amnesia and migraine. Ital J Neurol Sci. 1988;9:287–9.
63. Caplan L, Chedru F, Lhermitte F, Mayman C. Transient global amnesia and migraine. Neurology. 1981;31:1167–70.
64. Crowell GF, Stump DA, Biller J, McHenry LC Jr, Toole JF. The transient global amnesia-migraine connection. Arch Neurol. 1984;41:75–9.

65. Fernandez A, Rincon F, Mazer SP, Elkind MS. Magnetic resonance imaging changes in a patient with migraine attack and transient global amnesia after cardiac catheterization. CNS Spectr. 2005;10:980–3.
66. Olivarius BD, Jensen TS. Transient global amnesia in migraine. Headache. 1979;19:335–8.
67. Pradalier A, Lutz G, Vincent D. Transient global amnesia, migraine, thalamic infarct, dihydroergotamine, and sumatriptan. Headache. 2000;40:324–7.
68. Santoro G, Casadei B, Venco A. The transient global amnesia-migraine connection. Case Rep Funct Neurol. 1988;3:353–60.
69. Donnet A. Transient global amnesia triggered by migraine in a French tertiary-care center: an 11-year retrospective analysis. Headache. 2015;55:853–9.
70. Kimura S, Kumano T, Miyao S, Teramoto J. Herpes simplex encephalitis with transient global amnesia as an early sign. Intern Med. 1995;34:131–3.
71. McCorry DJ, Crowley P. Transient global amnesia secondary to herpes simplex viral encephalitis. Q J Med. 2005;98:154–5.
72. Fujimoto H, Imaizumi T, Nishimura Y, et al. Neurosyphilis showing transient global amnesia-like attacks and magnetic resonance imaging abnormalities mainly in the limbic system. Intern Med. 2001;40:439–42.
73. Pommer B, Pilz P, Harrer G. Transient global amnesia as a manifestation of Epstein-Barr virus encephalitis. J Neurol. 1983;229:125–7.
74. Daniel BT. Transient global amnesia. Print version and ebook: Amazon; 2012.
75. Hauge T. Catheter vertebral angiography. Acta Radiologica Suppl. 1954;109:1–219.
76. Duan H, Li L, Zhang Y, Zhang J, Chen M, Bao S. Transient global amnesia following neural and cardiac angiography may be related to ischemia. Biomed Res Int. 2016;2016:2821765.
77. Ghoneim MM. Transient global amnesia: a cause for postanesthetic memory disorder. Anesth Analg. 1998;87:980–1.
78. Bortolon RJ, Weglinski MR, Sprung J. Transient global amnesia after general anesthesia. Anesth Analg. 2005;101:916–9.
79. Graff-Radford J, Clapp AJ, Lanzino G, Rabinstein AA. Transient amnesia after coiling of a posterior circulation aneurysm. Neurocrit Care. 2013;18:245–7.
80. Lee BH. Transient global amnesia following carotid artery stenting: a case report. Radiol Case Rep. 2020;15:1159–63.
81. Baezner H, Blahak C, Capelle HH, Schrader C, Lutjens G, Krauss JK. Transient global amnesia associated with accidental high-frequency stimulation of the right hippocampus in deep brain stimulation for segmental dystonia. Stereotact Funct Neurosurg. 2013;91:335–7.
82. Profice P, Rizzello V, Pennestri F, et al. Transient global amnesia during transoesophageal echocardiogram. Neurol Sci. 2008;29:477–9.
83. Cassar MP, Balkhausen K. Transient global amnesia following transoesophageal echocardiography. BMJ Case Rep. 2020;13:e234751.
84. Cole AJ, Gloor P, Kaplan R. Transient global amnesia: the electroencephalogram at onset. Ann Neurol. 1987;22:771–2.
85. Hiraga A, Matsunaga T. Transient global amnesia and gastroscopy. J Neurol Neurosurg Psychiatry. 2006;77:995–6.
86. Neuzillet C, Merrouche M, Jouet P, Sabate JM, Coffin B. Transient global amnesia induced by esophageal functional exploration [in French]. Gastroenterol Clin Biol. 2009;33:1068–70.
87. Sayilir A, Kurt M, Ibis M, Kekilli M, Onal IK, Sasmaz N. Transient global amnesia following upper gastrointestinal endoscopy without premedication. Gastroenterol Nurs. 2009;32:362.
88. Ahn S, Kim W, Lee YS, et al. Transient global amnesia: seven years of experience with diffusion-weighted imaging in an emergency department. Eur Neurol. 2011;65:123–8.
89. Cesar S, Perdigao S. Transient global amnesia after gastroscopy. J Neurol. 2012;259(Suppl1):S140–1. (abstract P558)
90. Jeong M, Kim WS, Kim AR, Park JJ, Choi DH, Kim HY. Medical procedure-related transient global amnesia. Eur Neurol. 2018;80:42–9.

91. Benke T, Chemelli A, Lottersberger C, Waldenberger P, Karner E, Trinka E. Transient global amnesia triggered by the intracarotid amobarbital procedure. Epilepsy Behav. 2005;6:274–8.
92. Ravaglia S, Zito A, Ahmad L, Canavero I. How to forget a "traumatic" experience: a case report of transient global amnesia after nasopharyngeal swab for coronavirus disease 19. BMC Neurol. 2021;21:266.
93. Hirschfeld G, Sperfeld AD, Kassubek J, Scharffetter-Kochanek K, Sunderkotter C. Transient global amnesia (TGA) during an oral provocation test [in German]. Hautarzt. 2007;58:149–52.
94. Reinholz M, Heppt MV, Hoffmann FS, et al. Transient memory impairment and transient global amnesia induced by photodynamic therapy. Br J Dermatol. 2015;173:1258–62.
95. Robbins MS, Breidbart DH, Robbins HY. Transient global amnesia complicating pulmonary function testing. Respir Med CME. 2010;3:230–1.
96. Williamson JC, Larner AJ. Confused after spirometry: a unifying diagnosis. BMJ Case Rep. 2016;2016:pii:bcr2016216645.
97. Mokabberi R, Assal C, Afsaneh HM, Storm R, Dandamudi G. Transient global amnesia after ablation of premature ventricular beats arising from the right coronary cusp. Indian Pacing Electrophysiol J. 2010;10:372–5.
98. Park S, Park S, Jang Y. Transient global amnesia after stellate ganglion block. J Anesth. 2015;29:643.
99. Gomez-Choco M, Mariaca AF, Gaebel C, Valdueza JM. A controlled Valsalva maneuver causes neither diffusion-positive hippocampal lesions nor clinical symptoms after transient global amnesia. Eur Neurol. 2019;82:113–5.
100. Jeong M, Jin J, Kim JH, Moon Y, Choi JW, Kim HY. Incidental hippocampal hyperintensity on diffusion-weighted MRI: individual susceptibility to transient global amnesia. Neurologist. 2017;22:103–6.

Chapter 9
Pathogenesis of TGA

Abstract This chapter considers the pathogenesis of TGA, examining the evidence for and against the commonly considered possibilities, including cerebrovascular disease (arterial or venous), epilepsy and migraine. At time of writing, the pathogenesis of TGA remains enigmatic, and the possibility that this is a heterogeneous disorder cannot be excluded. Some possible applications of connectionist and computational neural network models to TGA pathogenesis and their mechanistic implications are considered.

Keywords TGA · Pathogenesis · Cerebrovascular disease · Epilepsy · Migraine · Genetics

9.1 What Is the Cause of TGA?

The pathogenesis of TGA remains unknown, although it has been much discussed in the six decades since the first clear descriptions of the condition [1–5]. It is not only a subject of interest to clinicians but also to patients and their relatives, who frequently pose the question at clinical consultation after the event.

Considering factors relevant to the epidemiology of TGA, the recognised predisposing (Chap. 7) and precipitating factors (Chap. 8) may give pointers to pathogenesis but without currently providing a compelling account of its origins.

Any pathogenetic theory faces a number of stern challenges to explain the empirically observed clinical and epidemiological features of TGA. It must take into account factors such as the very low frequency of recurrence (i.e. non-recurrence in the majority of cases), as well as the recognised predisposing and precipitating factors (at least the better established of these). Raymond Adams was of the view that "an explanation for episodic global amnesia must take into account the lack of morphologic change" (cited in [6], p.145).

It must also be borne in mind that the search for a unifying pathogenetic explanation for TGA, what might be described as the application of Ockham's (or Occam's) razor, may be a chimaera: as Caplan ([7], p.205) pointed out, TGA "might be caused by diverse processes sharing only a predilection for involvement of anatomical and physiological regions critical for memory registration and retrieval", hence different instances of TGA may simply be phenocopies of different disorders resulting from differing pathogenetic pathways. Roach argued for TGA as a symptom complex rather than a specific disease entity [8], and Quinette et al. thought TGA might refer to a single expression of several pathophysiological phenomena [9]. Certainly, some authors consider TGA to be a "heterogeneous disorder" ([10], p.188).

What strategies or investigations might be undertaken to elucidate TGA pathogenesis? The brevity and infrequency of episodes make investigations during the ictus difficult, but not impossible, as seen for a number of clinical investigations (as described in Chaps. 4 and 5). Traditionally, case–control studies and population-based studies have been used to try to address questions of disease aetiology, of which the latter are much preferred since they are free of many of the inherent biases of the former. Although numerous case–control studies of TGA have been reported (e.g. [11–18].), nationwide population-based cohort studies of TGA using large databases have only become available in recent times (e.g. [19–22].). Likewise, systematic reviews [23–27] and meta-analyses [26, 28, 29] of the evidence base in TGA are relatively recent.

A number of possibilities, sometimes referred to as theories or hypotheses, have repeatedly been advanced to try to explain TGA, including but not limited to: cerebrovascular disease (arterial or venous), epilepsy and migraine. These mirror to some extent the disorders with which TGA may be confused clinically and which enter the differential diagnosis (Chap. 3). Each of these possibilities is now considered, prior to an attempted formulation of the evidence.

9.2 Cerebrovascular Disease

9.2.1 Arterial

The abrupt onset of TGA may resemble that of a stroke or transient ischaemic attack (TIA). This has prompted considerations of transient arterial occlusion or cerebrovascular insufficiency as the causative factors for TGA from the time of the earliest descriptions, so much so that some authors were ready to classify TGA as a vascular phenomenon (e.g. [30–32].), a view which persisted in some quarters up until the 1990s [33]. Clinicians unfamiliar with TGA may still, not unreasonably, consider the possibility of stroke when they encounter patient with TGA [34]. Stroke mimicking TGA (i.e. "amnesic stroke") is uncommon but increasingly recognised with MR imaging studies (Sect. 3.1.2. and Table 3.4).

However, the evidence from prospective series of TGA cases is fairly conclusive that TGA does not share the same vascular risk factors as TIA (Sect. 7.11) and that there is no increased stroke risk at follow-up [19] although there is contradictory evidence [20] (Sect. 6.3.3). Such observations argue against a cerebrovascular aetiology, at least of thromboembolic origin: "there is no evidence to support thrombo-embolic disease as the cause of TGA in the majority of cases" ([35], p.137–8). Paradoxical embolism of platelet aggregates into the posterior cerebral circulation via a patent foramen ovale (PFO) is another suggested mechanism [36], but the evidence for an increased frequency of PFO in TGA patients is not compelling (Sect. 3.1.6).

The absence of thromboembolic risk factors does not necessarily preclude an arterial origin for TGA: some form of vasculopathy might also be implicated. Based on the association with migraine, Caplan et al. thought that "vascular spasm" might explain TGA in some patients, even those without evident migraine [37], and Caplan characterised the possible vascular changes as "acute arterial dyscontrol" [7].

The confident rejection of a cerebrovascular aetiology based on case–control studies comparing TGA and TIA cases was given pause with the findings of diffusion-weighted magnetic resonance imaging (MR-DWI) (Sect. 5.1.2; Fig. 5.1) showing transient signal changes evolving within the hippocampus, particularly the CA1 region, which were thought by some authors to be consistent with an ischaemic aetiology (Sect. 5.1.2.6). However, the frequency with which these imaging findings are seen seems to increase for the 2–3 days immediately post-event, unlike the findings in acute stroke, followed by resolution of the changes. This pattern has prompted some authors to suggest that TGA is not related to cerebral arterial ischaemia (e.g. [38].). Follow-up imaging to show persistence of changes is surely required to prove stroke as the aetiology of TGA (Sect. 3.2).

If these transient ischaemic signal changes within the hippocampus are not a consequence of vascular occlusion, then perhaps they might reflect enhanced vasoreactivity (Caplan's "acute arterial dyscontrol"?), with focal vasoconstriction inducing changes in the areas of the hippocampus, specifically CA1, known to be particularly vulnerable to ischaemia [39]. These changes might be of neurovascular origin, perhaps related to autonomic activation (a probable consequence or accompaniment of many of the recognised precipitating factors for TGA; Chap. 8), resulting in enhanced vasoreactivity and vasomotor instability/dysregulation. However, Baracchini et al. found no evidence for intracranial arterial vasoconstriction in TGA [40], although this does not necessarily indicate what is happening at capillary level within the hippocampal watershed.

9.2.2 Venous

Prompted in part by the inadequacy of other explanations for TGA, Lewis proposed that venous ischaemia in diencephalic or medial temporal lobe structures might be the cause of TGA. Noting that a Valsalva manoeuvre may be a factor common to many of the precipitating causes of TGA (Sect. 8.9), the argument was put forward that this might block venous return through the superior vena cava secondary to raised intrathoracic pressure, with retrograde transmission of high venous pressure into the cerebral venous system with resultant focal venous ischaemia [41].

Lewis's hypothesis has been influential and received a substantial boost with the consistent finding of internal jugular vein valve incompetence in greater frequency in TGA patients compared to controls (e.g. see the meta-analysis of Modabbernia et al. [29]; Sect. 4.3.3.2). This anatomical abnormality might be supposed to predispose to venous reflux, for example in association with a Valsalva manoeuvre, with resultant venous hypertension. Some authors have expressed strong support for a venous aetiology (e.g. [42, 43].). However, studies which have examined intracranial venous circulation in TGA have found little or no difference compared to controls (e.g. [44, 45].). Hence, the relevance of internal jugular vein valve incompetence to the pathogenesis of TGA remains uncertain [46]. Furthermore, the MR-DWI findings in TGA are said not to resemble venous congestion or infarcts [47]. Controlled Valsalva manoeuvre in patients with previous TGA produced no recurrence of symptoms or typical MR-DWI findings [48] (Sect. 8.9). Hence, at time of writing, Lewis's hypothesis is not proven.

Solheim and Skeidsvoll further developed the venous hypertension hypothesis by suggesting that most cases of TGA may be due to small thrombi in the deep cerebral venous system [49]. Although clinical reports of TGA in association with cerebral venous thrombosis are extremely rare (Sect. 3.1.4), Solheim and Skeidsvoll tried to pre-empt this objection by suggesting that small venous thrombi which are difficult to visualise with modern imaging technology may be responsible.

9.3   Epilepsy

The abrupt onset of TGA prompted consideration of an epileptic aetiology from the earliest studies [3, 4]:

> In our opinion the episodes, by virtue of their brevity, transiency, reversibility, and associated suspension of memory recording, bear a close resemblance to the amnesic spells described in temporal lobe seizures. … If the episodes are temporal lobe seizures, all prodromal and ictal phenomena other than the impairment of memory and possibly slight incoherence of thought were stripped away ([4], p.46).

A form of seizure affecting the hippocampal–diencephalic system remained Fisher's favoured explanation for TGA [50], notwithstanding the long duration of TGA attacks compared to most epileptic seizures. A form of non-convulsive status has been mooted, and the lack of EEG signature (Sects. 4.2.1 and 4.2.2) ascribed to the electrical changes occurring deep within the hippocampus and hence undetectable by traditional EEG methods.

Another stumbling block for the epilepsy hypothesis related to the usual single event phenotype of TGA, whilst epilepsy is usually recurrent, indeed this was one of the factors which helped to differentiate transient epileptic amnesia (TEA; Sect. 3.2.1) from TGA. Although an epileptic origin for TGA seems highly unlikely in the majority of cases, nonetheless TGA and TEA may not be mutually exclusive;

the possibility remains that there may be a pathogenetic interaction between them (Sect. 3.2.2).

Disturbances of brain electrical activity in a non-seizure form might still be pertinent to TGA pathogenesis, in the form of spreading depolarisation (Sect. 9.7.5).

9.4 Migraine

Many early authors posited a TGA-migraine connection (e.g. [37, 51, 52].) and this has been borne out by the high frequency of migraine consistently observed in series of patients with TGA, around one-third, (Sect. 7.9). The most reductive view is that "TGA is probably a migraine aura in most cases" ([53], p.125–30, 168).

Perhaps the strongest objection to this possible explanation of TGA pathogenesis is that migraine is generally understood as a recurrent condition whereas TGA is not, being a single event in most cases. That said, migraine can certainly manifest as an episode of transient amnesia (Sect. 3.4.1) which might be mistaken for TGA and hence may be included in the differential diagnosis, and as a precipitating event for TGA (Sect. 8.6).

If TGA is not migraine, nevertheless there is probably a link between the two conditions, as shown by the frequency of migraine in patients who have suffered from TGA (Sect. 7.9) and in familial cases of TGA (Sect. 7.8).

Patient age might also be relevant here. Clearly, TGA is more common with increasing age, at least until the seventh decade (see Sect. 7.4; Fig. 7.2), suggesting that the ageing brain is more vulnerable, and/or the younger brain is protected against or less susceptible, to whatever process(es) underpin(s) TGA. Migraine may manifest as a different phenotype in younger people, acute confusional migraine, which has been noted to have some similarities with TGA (Sects. 3.4.1 and 7.4). The paucity of reports of TGA after 80+ years may suggest that the oldest old brains may also be protected against TGA (Sect. 7.4). Of possible note, de novo presentation of migraine with aura in the eighth decade is unusual [54]. Primary headache associated with sexual activity (also known as coital cephalalgia), which is another acute neurological disorder related to sexual activity [55], also seems to show an increased incidence with age. Another possibility might be that TGA and migraine could be different phenotypic reflections of common underlying pathophysiological mechanisms, possibly related to particular genotypes.

As for TGA, the mechanisms underpinning migraine aura and headache remain a subject of debate, but the possible relevance of the neurophysiological process of cortical spreading depression (CSD), first described by Aristides Leão in 1944 [56] has been suggested, initially by Milner in 1958 [57] and then independently by Lauritzen [58] and Pearce [59], both in 1985. The possibility that hippocampal CSD might be a causative mechanism in TGA was first postulated by Olesen and Jorgensen in 1986 [60]. CSD is now characterised as part of the process of spreading depolarisation which is considered further in Sect. 9.7.5.

9.5   Genetics

The role of genetic factors in TGA pathogenesis has been relatively infrequently discussed because of the limited number of familial cases reported (see Sect. 7.8 and Table 7.3). However, some authors have explicitly questioned whether TGA might be genetic (e.g. [61, 62].), although clearly not a Mendelian disorder.

Given the infrequency of TGA, Arena and Rabinstein suggested that familial clusters may not be coincidental, and may possibly reflect a common genetic predisposition to migraine and TGA [63]. However, migraine was specifically mentioned in only a minority (16/53) of the familial cases reported in the literature (Sect. 7.8 and Table 7.3). This might simply represent incomplete reporting, although many of the studies were explicit about the absence of a migraine history (e.g. Case Study 7.1). In this context, Dupuis et al. reported (in abstract) a higher recurrence rate and history of migraine in those TGA patients with a positive family history of TGA (10 families) in a cohort of 219 patients seen over an extended period of time (1999–2016) [64]. The possible linkage of family history of TGA, migraine and recurrence merits further examination in large patient cohorts [65].

Another possibility might be that TGA and migraine could be different phenotypic reflections of common underlying pathophysiological mechanisms related to a particular genotype, or possibly to age: if childhood migraine may sometimes present as acute confusional migraine, it might be credible to argue that adult migraine (sometimes adult-onset migraine) might present as TGA (Sect. 9.4). The possible associations of TGA with psychological profile and psychiatric disorders on the anxiety–depression axis (Sect. 7.10) might also reflect shared pathophysiology, underpinned by polygenic mechanisms.

What genetic factors might be implicated? To date, genetic studies of TGA are few. Agosti et al. looked at the V66M polymorphism in the gene encoding brain-derived neurotrophic factor (BDNF) which had previously been demonstrated to affect human memory and hippocampal function in the development and maintenance of adult neurones. In a cohort of 98 TGA patients, there was no difference in the distribution of this BDNF genotype compared to controls [66]. This targeted approach to specific polymorphisms, although hypothesis-driven, is akin to searching for a needle in a haystack. Unbiased genome-wide association studies might potentially shed further light on any genetic factors which could be implicated in TGA pathogenesis.

Many paroxysmal neurological disorders have been found to be due to dysfunction of membrane ion channels [67], so the possibility that TGA might be a form of channelopathy seems a reasonable consideration. To date, I am not aware of any empirical evidence in favour of this possible explanation. Moreover, it is difficult to see why this explanation, as for stroke, epilepsy and migraine [67], would fit for a disorder usually characterised by single rather than recurrent events. Nevertheless, subtle changes in ion channel kinetics might contribute to TGA pathogenesis [68] (Sect. 9.7.5).

9.6 Psychiatry

The possibility that TGA might be a psychogenic disorder, explicable by "functional mechanisms", is mentioned here only to dismiss it. As previously described (Sect. 1.2), cases of possible TGA which predate the papers of Fisher and Adams [3, 4] might have been "immersed in the literature on psychogenic amnesia" ([35], p.4). Possible examples may be found in the publications of Kanzer (1939) [69] and Kennedy and Neville (1957) [70]. From the 1960s onwards, there was a decrease in reports of "hysterical amnesia".

Psychogenic amnesia is now conceptualised as a disorder distinct from TGA, although it enters the differential diagnosis (see Sect. 3.3). However, in view of the recognition of emotional factors as a frequent precipitating event for TGA (Sect. 8.1), it is not difficult to see why TGA might once have been considered a psychogenic disorder if onset was associated with evident psychological stresses [71]. Neurology is replete with disorders once thought to be psychiatric in origin (e.g. Tourette disorder, dystonia) now considered "organic".

9.7 Formulation: Towards a Neural Network Hypothesis

In the first edition of this book, some speculations as to the aetiopathogenesis of TGA were suggested but no hypothesis was attempted ([72], p.125–7). Although nothing in that general account now appears particularly objectionable or in need of refutation or withdrawal, the opportunity for further reflections has permitted the development of ideas and a tentative hypothesis of TGA pathogenesis based on neural network models. But before presenting these models, some consideration of existing models of TGA is in order.

9.7.1 Existing Models of TGA: Experimental and Theoretical

Whilst many models of memory and amnesia have been proposed, those specifically addressing TGA are few.

Considering experimental animal models, many have been developed in the investigation of the mechanisms underpinning amnesia, including transient amnesia (e.g. [73]). Although animal studies purporting to model aspects of TGA, specifically concurrent anterograde and retrograde amnesia, have been published [74, 75], to my knowledge these animal models have not been used to inform the understanding of TGA.

Experimental induction of TGA episodes in humans, which might permit in vivo studies, has been reported, but to my knowledge there are only two published examples, both unintentional. Moreover, the first of these reports can probably be discounted.

Castellani et al. [76] described a volunteer ("Subject 13") for an experiment examining the effects of repeated cold water (20 °C) immersion who, on a third exposure, developed "altered affect ... whimpering, anxious delirium-like state" for 20 min, of which he subsequently had no recollection. Despite the authors' statement that TGA is "typically 20 min in duration" ([76], p.154), this episode was in fact rather brief for such an attack, TGA rarely lasting less than 1 hour (Sect. 2.1.4). It was also atypical in the subject's age (23 years) and in the reported features, hence does not appear (retrospectively) to conform to suggested diagnostic criteria for TGA [77].

The second report described a 66-year-old patient with segmental dystonia which was treated with deep brain stimulation (DBS) of the globus pallidus interna. Baezner et al. reported that testing of one of the DBS electrodes, two years after implantation, at >6 V stimulation resulted in the patient questioning where she was and what was happening, with evidence of retrograde amnesia for the past few years, lasting for about 60 minutes. The stimulated electrode was found on subsequent MR brain imaging to have been misplaced in the right hippocampus [78]. The authors reported that all TGA criteria [77] were fulfilled and suggested that the stimulation procedure caused either "inhibition of local neuronal activity or fibre activation by high current density via direct electrical stimulation of hippocampal structures" ([78], p.336). Although too much weight should not be placed on single case studies, as they constitute the lowest (anecdotal) level of clinical evidence, the empirical observations reported by Baezner et al. might be pertinent to any proposed model of TGA pathogenesis. DBS may be characterised as creating "a virtual lesion by inducing electrophysiological silence in a neural circuit" and has even been suggested as a possible mechanism to erase memories ([79], p.120, 122).

Even if TGA could be reliably induced experimentally, there would be significant ethical questions to consider [79], the generally excellent prognosis of TGA notwithstanding (moreover, the prognosis of TGA, particularly if recurrent, may not be entirely benign; see Chap. 6).

Theoretical models of amnesia, as for experimental animal models, have been developed, but few specifically address TGA.

Meeter and Murre [80] developed the TraceLink model, inspired in part by David Marr's computational theory of archicortical function [81], to explain various forms of amnesia, in which the hippocampal complex was characterised as part of a link system involved in regulating its own plasticity through a modulating system. Simulation of TGA was achieved through suppressing any activity in the link layer, which showed both anterograde amnesia and temporally graded retrograde amnesia ([80], p.572–3 and Fig. 7). Gradual increase in link layer activity simulated the gradual lifting of TGA, with only amnesia for the pattern learned during the attack remaining thereafter, with resolution of all other amnesia. Based on their TraceLink model simulation of TGA, Meeter and Murre advanced an empirical claim that it should be possible to detect pathologically low activity level within the link system (i.e. medial temporal lobe structures) [80].

In the subsequent Memory Chain Model developed by Murre et al. [82], there was no explicit mention of TGA, although the retrograde amnesia in two TGA cases reported by Kritchevsky and Squire [83] (Sect. 4.1.1.3) was modelled ([82], p.13, and Table 3 rows o and p; and p.16, Fig. 13 plots o1,o2, p1, p2). In the discussion, it was reported that the expected lifetime of a single memory trace in the medial temporal lobe in TGA was 0.2–4 years, compared to 3–30 days from animal data ([82], p.16). No modelling or discussion of TGA anterograde amnesia was presented in this paper.

9.7.2   State-Transition Models

Because there is a finite probability of its recurrence (Sect. 6.2), TGA may be conceptualised using a simple state-transition type of Markov process which allows for repeated uncertain events. Two mutually exclusive clinical states are represented in the state-transition diagram (Fig. 9.1), TGA ("acute") and not-TGA (i.e. normal, or, because of the risk of repeated events, "dormant"). These might also be labelled, respectively, as hippocampal dysfunction and normal function. Patients are most likely to remain in the not-TGA (dormant) state over successive time periods. Since TGA events are not frequent, a cycle of 1 year has been used in the illustrated model, permitting use of empirically measured annual recurrence rates (Sect. 6.2.1) to denote the transition probabilities. As the patient is envisaged as being in one of two states and mortality is not involved, this is a non-absorbing model.

An implication of this modelling is that TGA is a stochastic process, evolving over time with associated uncertainty. Whether or not the behaviour of the process in any cycle is independent of the prior or future history of that cycle

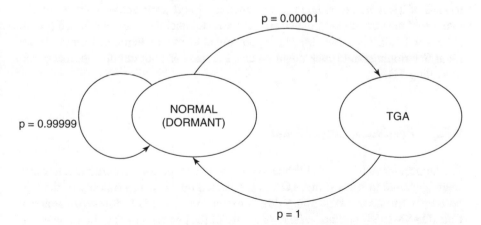

Fig. 9.1 State-transition diagram, or two-state Markov process. Numbers adjacent to arrows indicate probabilities of making that transition. The sum of the probabilities leading out of any state must be one

("memorylessness"), that being the restriction which defines a Markov process (Fig. 9.1 might also be described as illustrating a two-state Markov process), is uncertain for TGA (see discussion of recurrent TGA in Sect. 6.2.2). Clearly for other paroxysmal neurological events such as epilepsy or migraine, this "lack of memory" for the process does not hold. However, it remains possible that in TGA there is "memorylessness" for amnesia!

A rapid change in a network's connectivity, from local to global or vice versa, characterises phase transition. Such networks may be described using percolation theory as developed by Broadbent and Hammersley [84] and are subject to Kolmogorov's zero-one law such that an infinite network will have or not have (= probability one or zero) an infinite cluster. Hence, there is a percolation threshold, no matter what the shape of the network. Such networks are at risk of a sudden loss of connectivity. Based on these considerations, TGA might be envisaged as a consequence of a rapid phase transition in a neuronal network from normal to abnormal connectivity, specifically loss of connectivity, the threshold being variable between individuals (dependent upon their existing predisposing factors and susceptibility to precipitating factors). Unlike theoretical infinite networks, which have sharp phase transitions, such a real-world finite (and messy) network as the hippocampal formation would be anticipated to have more rounded transitions. At the cellular level, one might envisage that if hippocampal neurones become refractory for any reason, they might effectively drop out of the network which might eventually reach a threshold at which there is a sudden loss of connectivity.

Evidently, such state- or phase-transition models pay little, if any, attention to the underlying neurobiology of TGA (although Markov chains have been used to simulate neocortical function [85]). Along with the previously mentioned theoretical models (Sect. 9.7.1), they may be characterised as "top down" approaches, based on an attempt to model clinically observed phenomena. The general inadequacy of connectionist models in terms of biological plausibility suggests a need for further models of TGA based on large-scale dynamic circuit level analysis. Accordingly, two neural network models, which are not mutually exclusive, are postulated (Sects. 9.7.3 and 9.7.4). These are based on hippocampal formation neuroanatomy and neuronal functioning, and hence might be characterised as "bottom up" approaches to modelling TGA.

9.7.3   Feedback Loop Model

The hippocampus has an established role in memory function. Accordingly, it would seem plausible to suggest that TGA is predicated on the neuroanatomy of the hippocampal formation. Describing this neuroanatomy in 1911, Santiago Ramón y Cajal (1852–1934) outlined a functional circuit [86] which governs the direction of impulse flow through the hippocampal formation. This was also recognised in the later notion of a "trisynaptic circuit" [87] which, although now recognised to be an oversimplification, emphasised unidirectionality. Hippocampal anatomy is now characterised as a series of multiple, embedded loops (Fig. 9.2) which are briefly described here.

The hippocampal formation may be described as comprising a number of regions: the entorhinal cortex (EC), dentate gyrus (DG), subfields of the hippocampus proper denoted CA1 and CA3 (nomenclature derived from the work of Lorente de Nó, [88], one of Cajal's pupils) and the subiculum. CA3 is the major input to CA1 via the collaterals first described by, and now named for, Schaffer [89]. CA1 projects to the subiculum (Sub), and both CA1 and Sub project to EC, with CA1 axons returning to the same EC region from which they receive their input. A projection from the deep to the superficial layers of the EC completes the closed loop [90]. The outputs of the hippocampal formation are via the Sub and EC, respectively mainly subcortical (via the fimbria–fornix pathway) and cortical projections.

Hence, a long loop runs from EC via the perforant path (PP) to DG and then to the subfields of the hippocampus proper, with output via Sub and/or EC. As EC receives inputs from many areas of associative neocortex (parietal, prefrontal, temporal) via the parahippocampal gyrus and perirhinal cortex, this pathway funnels highly processed multimodal sensory information into the hippocampal formation. DG granule cells project mossy fibre axons to the CA3 field pyramidal cells. DG is recognised to have a gating function [91], filtering afferent inputs to the hippocampus proper (CA3), thus enacting a sparse coding scheme which permits overlapping

Fig. 9.2 Simple schematic block diagram representation of the major pathways of signal flow from cortex to hippocampal formation and back to cortex, showing embedded hippocampal loops. *PP,* perforant path; *MF,* mossy fibres; *TA,* temporoammonic pathway; *A/C,* associative/commissural loop; *SC,* Schaffer collaterals

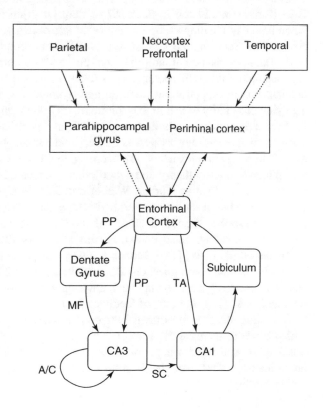

or very similar inputs to the hippocampus to be separated from one another, the process of pattern separation, and hence many different memories to be encoded and stored.

In addition to the long loop, an intermediate loop runs from EC directly to CA3 via PP, hence to CA1, Sub and/or EC; whilst a short loop runs directly from EC to CA1 via the temporoammonic projection (TA) running in the alvear pathway, hence to Sub and/or EC. There are no immediate reciprocal connections to preceding regions (i.e. no projection of DG to EC, of CA3 to DG or of CA1 to CA3).

CA3 receives not only the aforementioned mossy fibre inputs from DG and a direct PP projection from EC but also has recurrent collateral connections extending throughout CA3, sometimes known as the associative/commissural (A/C) loop. These latter connections far outnumber PP and DG mossy fibre inputs to CA3 (in the rat, 12,000, vs 3600 and 46, respectively, per CA3 cell). CA3 may thus be a final convergence point for inputs from DG mossy fibres, EC and CA3 recurrent collaterals.

In addition to the excitatory connections, there are also inhibitory connections within the hippocampal formation (not shown in Fig. 9.2), both feedforward (DG to CA3 interneurons to CA3 pyramidal cells) and feedback (CA3 pyramidal cells to CA3 interneurons).

The operation of these hippocampal CA3 circuits is considered to be central to memory encoding and recall [92]. The recurrent, autoassociative connections of CA3 (further considered in Sect. 9.7.4) may underpin the retrieval of memories when inputs to the hippocampus are incomplete or degraded, the process of pattern completion. Such an autoassociative network is not found in CA1.

The characterisation of multiple loops embedded within the neuroanatomy of the hippocampal formation prompts consideration of the possible role of feedback mechanisms in hippocampal function and dysfunction. The concept of feedback, implying circularity of action, has a long history and many recognised applications in diverse disciplines, including mechanical and electrical engineering, chemistry, economics, meteorology, as well as biology and human physiology. Feedback loops are a feature of complex adaptive systems, and feedback is a central concept in the disciplines of control theory and cybernetics, pioneered in the 1940s and 1950s by mathematicians such as Norbert Wiener and John von Neumann. These interests extended to other disciplines including biology, and it may be noted that Lorente de Nó, who described the fine anatomy of the hippocampus [88], attended the early cybernetics meetings (also known as the Macy Foundation meetings) with von Neumann ([93], p.188; [94]). Morris Bender, one of the first clinicians to describe TGA, also attended as a guest on one occasion ([94], p.286), but I am not aware of any evidence to suggest he may have envisaged the "isolated episode of confusion with amnesia" [1, 2] in terms of feedback loops.

A distinction may be drawn between negative, or self-correcting, feedback, which tends to increase the stability and accuracy of operation of a system; and positive, or self-reinforcing, compounding or exacerbating, feedback in which amplification rather than stabilisation occurs but which risks exponential growth and instability.

Generally, negative feedback is a characteristic of purposeful or goal-directed actions or behaviours wherein error-signal controlled regulation typically involves integration causing asymptotic or oscillatory behaviour. In contrast, positive feedback systems tend to show exponential behaviour and hence achieve signal amplification, but the process is liable to collapse if unchecked and may risk being detrimental to the system. Generally, some form of negative feedback kicks in sooner or later to curtail unchecked positive feedback.

Negative and positive feedback may be characterised in terms of reduced or increased loop gain (= output/input) respectively. A feedback loop may be represented by a simple schematic block diagram (Fig. 9.3) where A and β represent arbitrary causal links or relations which denote the flow of causality (A = open-loop gain; β = feedback factor). The overall or closed-loop gain, G_c, may be expressed as:

$$G_c = A / (1 + \beta A)$$

where βA = loop gain. Hence, if $\beta = 0$ (i.e. no feedback), then product $\beta A = 0$, and so $G_c = A$ (i.e. open-loop gain). If $\beta A > 0$, then as $(1 + \beta A) > A$, there is negative feedback from input to output. If $\beta A < 0$, then as $(1 + \beta A) < A$, a positive feedback from input to output occurs. As βA approaches -1, the gain may be very large, an asymptotic increase typical of a reciprocal function. If $\beta A = -1$, then $(1 + \beta A) = 0$, so $G_c = A/0$, infinite gain. In this circumstance, a "runaway" situation will develop. For any function $f(x) = 1/x$, $x = 0$ corresponds to a discontinuity or singularity where the function "explodes" to $+/- \infty$ and so is not defined.

Might these feedback concepts be applicable to hippocampal function? Hebb characterised short-term memory as a reverberation of the closed loop of hippocampal cell assemblies [95], and negative feedback was an integral component of Marr's computational theory of archicortical function [81] (although the understanding of hippocampal neuroanatomy was somewhat different at the time Marr was writing).

If, based on its particular neuroanatomy, the hippocampal formation is characterised at the neural network level as a system of multiple, embedded loops, a feedback

Fig. 9.3 Simple schematic block diagram representation of a feedback loop. A = open-loop gain; β = feedback factor. Closed-loop gain $G_c = A/(1 + \beta A)$

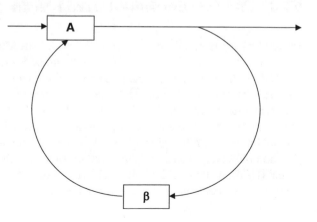

loop model of TGA pathophysiology may be envisaged. The proposed chain of causation is as follows.

Changes in the internal and external environment, the recognised precipitating factors of TGA (e.g. emotional, physical stressors; Chap. 8), lead to changes in interoceptive and exteroceptive signalling which converge on EC from association cortices. These increased inputs, perhaps acting on a predisposed system (as evidenced by, for example, an underlying migraine tendency, or genetic predisposition from a family history of TGA; Chap. 7), result in increased activation through the rest of the hippocampal formation. This might occur in various ways, involving the long, intermediate and/or short hippocampal formation loops. Specifically, opening of the dentate gate (i.e. less filtering) with repeated stimulation [91]; increased transmission through the TA pathway from EC to CA1; and/or enhanced autoassociation in CA3 recurrent collaterals (see Fig. 9.2). Positive feedback in any or all of the embedded loops would lead to amplified, neural firing, exacerbated if there were concurrent impairment or failure of inhibitory mechanisms (negative feedback from inhibitory interneurons) to stabilise inputs to the hippocampal closed-loop circuits. If gain within any or all of the loops becomes infinite, runaway neural firing results in a singularity or discontinuity: there is failure of synaptic transmission around the circuit, or elements thereof, with consequent failure of hippocampal mnestic functions, manifest clinically as the anterograde and retrograde amnesia typical of an episode of TGA. The duration of the TGA episode is then determined by the time required for the refractory system to re-establish normal synaptic transmission through the feedback circuit (see Sect. 9.7.5 for a consideration of pathogenic mechanisms).

Of course, this feedback loop model of TGA has limitations. Whilst simple systems may be described as exemplars of either negative or positive feedback, this categorisation may not be so easily established in the presence of multiple loops. Complex systems, wherein the loops are not independent (i.e. non-linear), may have complex behaviours and may best be treated as a whole.

9.7.4   CA3 Autoassociative Attractor Model

Inspired by the work of Brindley (1969) [96] and of Marr (1971) [81], and by the first analysis for operation of a synaptic network of Barlow and Levick (1965) [97], Bennett et al. suggested that the CA3 pyramidal neuronal connections formed an autoassociative network [98]. The random connections of CA3 neurones through recurrent collaterals were envisaged as the neuroanatomical substrate for the retrieval of memories under specific conditions. (Note that, in light of the application of linguistic philosophical considerations, discussed by Bennett and Hacker [99] and ultimately dating to Wittgenstein, Bennett subsequently reinterpreted his model ([100], p.106–7,112,114)). Following this, CA3 has been characterised as a single, global autoassociative attractor network [101].

Attractor networks, based on the cortical anatomy of recurrent collateral excitatory synaptic connections between pyramidal neurones, may constitute a funda-
mental principle of cerebral cortical function. This architecture has been used to
develop computational models of attentional, perceptual, mnestic and decision-
making functions and has also prompted predictions about impaired function in
certain clinical disorders of the brain [101–104].

In a simple attractor network (Fig. 9.4), external inputs to neurones, e_i, produce
output (postsynaptic) firing, r_i. Through recurrent collateral synapses, w_{ij}, e_i is associated with itself through presynaptic firing, r_j. Associative learning results in a
change in synaptic weight, δw_{ij}, dependent on pre- and postsynaptic firing:

$$\delta w_{ij} = k.r_i.r_j$$

where k is a constant. The network behaves probabilistically, influenced by the
strength of inputs, settling in a stable fixed attractor state or, in terms of an energy
landscape, basin of attraction: either a spontaneous low firing rate state, or one or
more persistent high firing rate states, respectively shallower or deeper basins of
attraction.

Positive feedback is inherent to the operation of attractor networks, implemented
through the recurrent collateral connections. The risk of exponential growth and
instability, with runaway neural firing, is prevented in the attractor network by the
non-linear activation function of neurones, such that they function in a binary (i.e.
firing or non-firing) rather than a continuously graded (linear) mode. The threshold
is set in part by negative feedback from inhibitory interneurons.

In the particular case of the CA3 autoassociative attractor network, positive feedback via recurrent collateral connections between CA3 pyramidal neurones can sus-
tain persistent neuronal firing, thus implementing different memories. Because of

Fig. 9.4 Autoassociative
attractor network

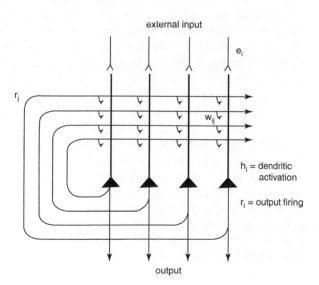

the widespread nature of the CA3 recurrent collateral connections, there is a fair chance that any one set of active neurones may be associated with any other set, these arbitrary associations forming a potential mechanism for implementing the different aspects of an episodic memory. CA3 attractor dynamics determine whether a new memory is stored, as a consequence of pattern separation with formation of a new basin of attraction, or an existing memory is retrieved, as a consequence of pattern completion and reactivation of an existing basin of attraction. Recoding in CA1 of information from CA3 is proposed to set up associatively learned back projections to the neocortex, itself modelled as multiple local attractor networks, based on the local recurrent collateral connections of neocortical pyramidal cells, to allow subsequent retrieval of information.

Applications of attractor theory to explain certain neurological and psychiatric diseases, such as obsessive-compulsive disorder, schizophrenia and depression, have been presented ([103], p.305–35). In addition, age-related impairments of episodic memory have been characterised as a reduction in the depth, and hence stability, of the basins of attraction of hippocampal attractor memory-related networks ([103], p.335–43; [104]). These conceptualisations might be extended to the case of TGA.

If, based on its neuroanatomy, hippocampal CA3 is characterised at the neural network level as a single global autoassociative attractor network, a model of TGA pathophysiology may be suggested [105]. The proposed chain of causation is as follows.

Positive feedback through the recurrent collateral CA3 connections becomes excessive as a consequence of changes in interoceptive and exteroceptive signalling converging on EC from association cortices, related to the recognised precipitating and predisposing factors for TGA (emotional stress, physical effort, etc.). There is enhanced activation of CA3 pyramidal cells via PP and DG inputs from EC to CA3 (Fig. 9.5). The binary mode functioning of CA3 neurones (firing or not firing) consequent upon their non-linear activation function renders them susceptible to not firing due to changes in threshold, related to concurrent impaired negative feedback from CA3 inhibitory interneurons. A runaway situation with infinite gain in the short CA3 feedback loop develops, resulting in a singularity or discontinuity, with failure of synaptic transmission (these steps overlap with those outlined in the feedback loop model in Sect. 9.7.3).

In terms of the attractor schematic (Fig. 9.4), postsynaptic firing, r_i, tends to zero, and hence the change in synaptic weight, δw_{ij}, also tends to zero. With no change in synaptic weights, no encoding of new memories or reactivation of existing memories within the hippocampus can occur. With loss of the output (CA3) neuronal firing (r_i), the network cannot compensate. There is loss of fault tolerance, one of the recognised properties of attractor networks, with catastrophic collapse of function, rather than the graceful degradation (proneness to error) anticipated with increased noise in a neural network, as may occur in age-related episodic memory impairment or Alzheimer's disease. In terms of the energy landscape, the system is unstable and flips to a shallower basin of attraction.

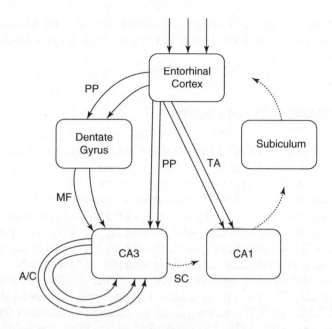

Fig. 9.5 Detail from Fig. 9.2 showing proposed hypothesis of TGA pathogenesis: excessive positive feedback in A/C loop following increased neocortical input to entorhinal cortex causes functional ablation of CA3 and failure of onward synaptic transmission to CA1 and neocortex. *PP*, perforant path; *MF*, mossy fibres; *TA*, temporoammonic pathway; *A/C*, associative/commissural loop; *SC*, Schaffer collaterals

Inactivation of the hippocampal CA3 attractor network accounts for inability to encode new associations (anterograde amnesia) and to retrieve some existing memories (retrograde amnesia). In addition to impaired recognition memory (pattern completion), evidence for impairment of pattern separation during acute TGA has been presented [106].

The consequent failure of feedforward excitation of CA1 from CA3, and hence of back projections to the neocortex from CA1 (Fig. 9.5), may also contribute to the failure to retrieve previously learned information, hence contributing to the retrograde amnesia (and possibly explaining its variable duration).

The intrinsic indeterminacy of attractor networks may also have some mechanistic corollaries of clinical relevance to TGA. Because of the stochastic operation of autoassociative attractor networks (as in the state-transition model; Sect. 9.7.2), it might be predicted that some TGA episodes may occur without obvious precipitants or triggers, but as a consequence of an inherently noisy system (possibly related to predisposing factors) flipping to a spontaneous low firing rate state as the most stable basin of attraction in the energy landscape.

Interindividual variation in the stability of the global CA3 attractor network may render some individuals at greater risk of episodes of TGA and their recurrence.,

This vulnerability might be structural or physiological, perhaps related to developmentally defined alterations in brain networks [68] or subtle variations in ion channel kinetics. Genetically determined factors may also be relevant, such as migraine tendency and/or family history of TGA, putting these individuals at greater risk of TGA.

9.7.5   Spreading Depolarisation

The feedback loop and CA3 autoassociative attractor models (Sects. 9.7.3 and 9.7.4) of TGA may be predicated on hippocampal anatomy and function, but what mechanism(s) might underpin these neural network models?

As previously mentioned in the context of migraine (Sect. 9.4), Olesen and Jorgensen suggested more than 30 years ago that the cortical spreading depression (CSD) first described by Leão [56] was "theoretically … a very likely pathogenetic mechanism of TGA", and more specifically that "A highly emotional experience excites the hippocampus. Neuronal activity liberates glutamate, which triggers a spreading depression resulting in reversible functional ablation of the hippocampus" ([60], p.220). The initial observations of hippocampal changes on MR-DWI in TGA (Sect. 5.1.2; Fig. 5.1) were interpreted as evidence in favour of a CSD mechanism in TGA (e.g. [107, 108]). The mechanism of spreading depression remains a potential candidate explanation for TGA [109]. A revision of this suggestion may align with the postulated neural network models of TGA pathogenesis.

Spreading depression is now characterised as part of a continuum with spreading depolarisation (SD). SD is a wave of electrophysiological hyperactivity followed by a wave of inhibition which propagates across the cerebral cortex at around 1–10 mm/min. SD may be triggered by different processes, including severe ischaemia, hypoxia, hypoglycaemia and epileptic events. SD is thought to disrupt neuronal electrical activity through changes in extracellular ion concentrations, particularly increased $[K^+]$, toxic release of glutamate, dispersion of electrochemical gradients (failure of Na^+/K^+-ATPase pumps), mitochondrial dysfunction and cytotoxic oedema, leading to prolonged neuronal membrane depolarisation and refractoriness to neuronal impulse and synaptic transmission (for more detail on SD, see reviews [110–112]).

Extracellular glutamate accumulation may exacerbate neuronal depolarisation via glutamate receptors, a further positive feedback loop. NMDA receptors, with their high conductance and slow kinetics compared to AMPA receptors, may be particularly significant. In simulations of attractor dynamics, relatively small changes in NMDA receptor conductance can result in reduced firing rate, synaptic strength, basin depth and signal-to-noise ratio [101]. With the gradual restoration of ionic electrochemical gradients through the action of energy-dependent ion pumps, which also promote glutamate uptake, neuronal membranes repolarise and synaptic transmission resumes. This restoration may correlate with recovery from the clinical episode of TGA and resumption of episodic memory function.

SD is recognised to be a heterogeneous entity, the exact nature of which is affected by the triggering event and by genetic background. It has been implicated in various disease processes, including stroke, traumatic brain injury, epileptic seizures and sudden unexplained death in epilepsy, as well as migraine aura, but recent reviews of SD do not mention, other than in passing, the previously postulated role in TGA. Many of the proposed mechanisms of SD are shared with epileptic seizures and ischaemia [113], but their occurrence in a hippocampal formation with essentially normal synaptic structure and perfusion may result in no significant long-term structural change. The vascular response to SD is variable, including both vasoconstriction and vasodilation. This might account for some of the variability in the changes in brain diffusivity seen on MR-DWI in TGA.

If SD is a "universal principle" of lesion development ([112], p.1572), it may be that TGA is a symptom complex which occurs as a consequence of SD. Current understandings of the pathogenesis of TGA (epilepsy, stroke, migraine) may not necessarily be mutually exclusive, indeed might be reconciled by the mechanisms of SD. For example, the TGA-migraine link may indicate a shared susceptibility to SD.

If the TGA rubric encompasses different entities, with TGA being a symptom complex [8] rather than a single specific disease entity, this might explain contradictory findings of epidemiological studies on factors such as the presence or absence of particular vascular risk factors. SD has also been proposed as an explanatory mechanism for seizures following migraine (migralepsy) and for migraine stroke or migrainous infarction [114].

9.7.6 Hypothesis: Proposal, Evidence, Predictions and Shortcomings

Could the proposed models of TGA, in particular the CA3 autoassociative attractor neural network catastrophic degradation model (Sect. 9.7.4), and the mechanism of spreading depolarisation (Sect. 9.7.5) be developed into a hypothesis of TGA pathogenesis which has an evidential basis and can make testable, falsifiable, predictions?

The hypothesis for the CA3 autoassociative attractor model may be stated as follows [105]. Proposal: An episode of TGA results when excessive positive feedback through the short recurrent collateral loops in the hippocampal CA3 region causes a temporary functional ablation of an autoassociative attractor neural network, flipping it to a spontaneous low firing rate state as the most stable basin of attraction in the energy landscape. Mechanistically, this is caused by a wave of spreading depolarisation which results in a cascade of biochemical and biophysical changes which produce prolonged neuronal membrane depolarisation and refractoriness to neuronal impulse and synaptic transmission, manifest clinically as the episode of anterograde and (variable) retrograde amnesia.

Some existing evidence may be deemed consistent with this hypothesis. Reports of functional neuroimaging studies, almost invariably undertaken post-TGA, have generally shown hypoperfusion (SPECT) and hypometabolism (PET) in and beyond medial temporal lobe structures (Sect. 5.2.1 and 5.2.2), but these imaging modalities are known to have low spatial resolution. Resting-state functional MR imaging has shown reduction in functional connectivity within the episodic memory network bilaterally during TGA, including but not limited to the hippocampus, and more evident in the hyperacute phase and fully reversible with time (Sect. 5.2.6). Unintentional induction of TGA when testing deep brain stimulation electrodes, found on subsequent MR brain imaging to have been misplaced in the right hippocampus, was interpreted as caused by either inhibition of local neuronal activity or fibre activation by high current density via direct electrical stimulation of hippocampal structures [78] (Sect. 9.7.1).

Evidence which may falsify, rather than verify, a hypothesis is acknowledged to be the most stringent test, as any hypothesis that cannot be rejected is outside the realm of the empirical. Studying TGA in vivo is difficult since experience indicates that opportunities are few and of relatively brief duration (e.g. [115].). Hence, any falsifiable clinical predictions of the hypothesis would be difficult to test logistically. The most parsimonious test would be to look for changes consistent with SD in the hippocampal CA3 region during a TGA episode, since its absence would falsify the hypothesis. However, clinical monitoring of SD is currently limited to the use of subdural electrode strips placed by highly invasive neurosurgical intervention [116]. This ultimate test of the hypothesis must await the development of other, less invasive, technologies which can reliably detect SD in vivo.

The rostrocaudal extent of the hippocampal formation is about 5 cm in length, and hence SD, propagating at 1–10 mm/min, would be anticipated to progress through it in about 5–50 min, too short a time to be observed by any investigative modality unless by extreme chance a patient developed TGA whilst in close proximity to suitable equipment. Were that to be the case, then powerful structural imaging, for example with 7 Tesla MR, might be predicted to detect the acute changes of cytotoxic oedema which typically accompany SD within the hippocampus (follow-up 7 T MR imaging studies of TGA showed no visible sequelae [117]). Other investigational options might include magnetoencephalography (MEG) to image hippocampal activity [118] or high-resolution MR spectroscopy [119]. AC/DC-EEG to measure propagated negative DC potentials, which are thought to be markers of SD, might also be used [120].

In addition to clinical investigations during an episode of TGA, testable predictions at the epidemiological level may be made in light of the hypothesis. For example, SD is recognised to reduce seizure threshold [111]. If this were the case following TGA, patients might be predicted to have increased vulnerability to the emergence of epileptic seizures. There is some tentative evidence in favour of this (see Sect. 6.3.4 for summary). Instances of TEA following TGA (Sect. 3.2.2) in association with medial temporal lobe structural abnormalities on standard MR imaging sequences might also be taken as support for the prediction of the hypothesis.

The proposed hypothesis is, of course, not without shortcomings. Two particular limitations may be highlighted: firstly the observed age-related incidence of TGA

(Sect. 7.4) and secondly the MR-DWI findings (Sect. 5.1.2). The increasing incidence of TGA with age might be explicable in terms of aging-related vulnerability of the hippocampal attractor network to noise-related instability, as for aging-related decline in episodic memory ([103], p.335–43; [104]), but the apparent decline in TGA incidence in the latest decades of life would not be predicted by this mechanism. This might possibly be an artefact of case underascertainment and/or underreporting of TGA in the very elderly. If genuine, it might be related to declining susceptibility of the brain to SD with age [121]. A lower experimental threshold for SD induction in females [111] might be consistent with the female preponderance seen in most TGA cohorts [26] (Sect. 7.5).

The MR-DWI neuroimaging findings suggesting the evolution of neuronal metabolic stress in CA1 elude definitive explanation, although might be a consequence of enhanced transmission through the direct TA pathway from EC to CA1. The variable vascular response to SD may also be relevant. The time course with which these imaging changes evolve suggests they may be downstream and non-specific events [122], a transient diaschisis related to the relative vulnerability of the CA1 hippocampal sector to hypoxic and ischaemic insults which has long been recognised [123, 124] and may perhaps be a consequence of mitochondrial dysfunction [125]. Notwithstanding the neuroimaging findings, the suggested model does not envisage TGA to be simply a consequence of a lesion or lesions restricted to CA1 (see also Sect. 5.1.2.6).

9.8 The Future?

How might the understanding of TGA be taken forward in the coming years? One might anticipate developments both at the individual and epidemiological levels.

At the individual level, investigation of patients in the acute phase of TGA using neuroradiological and neurophysiological methods of increasing sophistication might shed further light on pathogenesis (Sect. 9.7.6). This poses significant logistical challenges, including transporting patients to hospital as soon as possible after onset of TGA and provision of suitable facilities for assessment and investigation in emergency care or acute neurology settings. Addressing some of these challenges might be facilitated by awareness raising measures delivered to both clinicians and the general populace. However, since the most significant elements of TGA pathogenesis (e.g. spreading depolarisation) may predate clinical mnestic and behavioural symptomatology, even this may not be sufficient for meaningful investigation of pathogenesis, since by the time of assessment only downstream events might be accessible to study. Remote monitoring of patients susceptible to recurrent TGA, if these could be identified (Sect. 6.2.2), might address this, if suitable technology could be developed (the neuronal equivalent of a cardiac loop recorder?) and patients could be persuaded to accept its use.

To better understand possible predisposing factors such as age, gender, ethnicity, and history of migraine and psychiatric/psychological disorders, as well as precipitating factors, further large epidemiological studies of TGA are required. Ideally, such studies should be population-based to avoid bias. Ideally, there should be a minimum dataset collected for each patient, inquiring about pertinent clinical issues. Further consideration may need to be given to revising the Hodges and Warlow (1990) diagnostic criteria for TGA [77] to include MR-DWI (as has been previously suggested, e.g. [126]., p.109; see Sect. 2.2.2) to ensure relatively homogeneous patient cohorts and to exclude TGA mimics. Unbiased genome-wide association studies based on patients recruited to such studies, as well as metabolomic studies, might potentially shed further light on factors involved in TGA pathogenesis.

It may eventually be possible to move beyond purely descriptive neuroscience. As understanding of brain functional mechanisms develops, it may become possible to undertake computer-modelling of normal and pathological hippocampal neuronal network functions, perhaps using simulations of models such as those suggested here (Sects. 9.7.2, 9.7.3, and 9.7.4). By factoring in changes such as spreading depolarisation, it may be possible to see if TGA-like changes can be reproduced.

9.9   Closing Summary

Although much has been learned about TGA in the six decades since its first clear description, much still remains to be learned. The enigma of TGA pathogenesis will undoubtedly continue to intrigue clinicians and neuroscientists, and prompt further studies of this fascinating symptom complex/condition, not only because of its clinical significance but also because of the light it may shed on the cognitive architecture and mechanisms of human memory.

References

1. Bender MB. Syndrome of isolated episode of confusion with amnesia. J Hillside Hosp. 1956;5:212–5.
2. Bender MB. Single episode of confusion with amnesia. Bull NY Acad Med. 1960;36:197–207.
3. Fisher CM, Adams RD. Transient global amnesia. Trans Am Neurol Assoc. 1958;83:143–6.
4. Fisher CM, Adams RD. Transient global amnesia. Acta Neurol Scand. 1964;40(Suppl9):1–81.
5. Guyotat MM, Courjon J. Les ictus amnésiques. J Med Lyon. 1956;37:697–701.
6. Laureno R. Raymond Adams. A life of mind and muscle. Oxford: Oxford University Press; 2009.
7. Caplan LB. [sic]. Transient global amnesia. In: Frederiks JAM, editor. Handbook of clinical neurology. Volume 1 (45). Clinical neuropsychology. Amsterdam: Elsevier Science Publishers; 1985. p. 205–18.
8. Roach ES. Transient global amnesia: look at mechanisms not causes. Arch Neurol. 2006;63:1338–9.
9. Quinette P, Guillery-Girard B, Dayan J, de la Sayette V, Marquis S, Viader F, Desgranges B, Eustache F. What does transient global amnesia really mean? Review of the literature and thorough study of 142 cases. Brain. 2006;129:1640–58.

10. Pearce JMS, Bogousslavsky J. "Les ictus amnésiques" and transient global amnesia. Eur Neurol. 2009;62:188–92.
11. Guidotti M, Anzalone N, Morabito A, Landi G. A case-control study of transient global amnesia. J Neurol Neurosurg Psychiatry. 1989;52:320–3.
12. Hodges JR, Warlow CP. The aetiology of transient global amnesia. A case-control study of 114 cases with prospective follow-up. Brain. 1990;113:639–57.
13. Jang JW, Park SY, Hong JH, Park YH, Kim JE, Kim S. Different risk factor profiles between transient global amnesia and transient ischemic attack: a large case-control study. Eur Neurol. 2014;71:19–24.
14. Melo TP, Ferro JM, Ferro H. Transient global amnesia. A case control study. Brain. 1992;115:261–70.
15. Moreno-Lugris XC, Martinez-Alvarez J, Branas F, Martinez-Vazquez F, Cortes-Laino JA. Transient global amnesia. Case-control study of 24 cases [in Spanish]. Rev Neurol. 1996;24:554–7.
16. Schmidtke K, Ehmsen L. Transient global amnesia and migraine. A case control study. Eur Neurol. 1998;40:9–14.
17. Toledo M, Pujadas F, Purroy F, Lara N, Quintana M, Alvarez-Sabin J. Recurrent transient global amnesia, a manifestation of ischemic cerebrovascular disease [in Spanish]. Med Clin (Barc). 2005;125:361–5. [Erratum Med Clin (Barc). 2006;126:316]
18. Zorzon M, Antonutti L, Mase G, Biasutti E, Vitrani B, Cazzato G. Transient global amnesia and transient ischemic attack. Natural history, vascular risk factors, and associated conditions. Stroke. 1995;26:1536–42.
19. Garg A, Limaye K, Shaban A, Adams HP Jr, Leira EC. Transient global amnesia does not increase the risk of subsequent ischemic stroke: a propensity score-matched analysis. J Neurol. 2021;268:3301–6.
20. Lee SH, Kim KY, Lee JW, Park SJ, Jung JM. Risk of ischaemic stroke in patients with transient global amnesia: a propensity-matched cohort study. Stroke Vasc Neurol. 2021; https://doi.org/10.1136/svn-2021-001006. svn-2021-001006. Online ahead of print
21. Lin KH, Chen YT, Fuh JL, et al. Migraine is associated with a higher risk of transient global amnesia: a nationwide cohort study. Eur J Neurol. 2014;21:718–24.
22. Yi M, Sherzai AZ, Ani C, Shavlik D, Ghamsary M, Lazar E, Sherzai D. Strong association between migraine and transient global amnesia: a national inpatient sample analysis. J Neuropsychiatry Clin Neurosci. 2019;31:43–8.
23. Liampas I, Raptopoulou M, Mpourlios S, et al. Factors associated with recurrent transient global amnesia: systematic review and pathophysiological insights. Rev Neurosci. 2021;32:751–65.
24. Liampas I, Raptopoulou M, Siokas V, et al. Conventional cardiovascular risk factors in transient global amnesia: systematic review and proposition of a novel hypothesis. Front Neuroendocrinol. 2021;61:100909.
25. Liampas I, Raptopoulou M, Siokas V, et al. The long-term prognosis of transient global amnesia: a systematic review. Rev Neurosci. 2021;32:531–43.
26. Lim SJ, Kim M, Suh CH, Kim SY, Shim WH, Kim SJ. Diagnostic yield of diffusion-weighted brain magnetic resonance imaging in patients with transient global amnesia: a systematic review and meta-analysis. Korean J Radiol. 2021;22:1680–9.
27. Milburn-McNulty P, Larner AJ. Transient global amnesia and brain tumour: chance concurrence or aetiological association? Case report and systematic literature review. Case Rep Neurol. 2015;7:18–25.
28. Jäger T, Bazner H, Kliegel M, Szabo K, Hennerici MG. The transience and nature of cognitive impairments in transient global amnesia: a meta-analysis. J Clin Exp Neuropsychol. 2009;31:8–19.
29. Modabbernia A, Taslimi S, Ashrafi M, Modabbernia MJ, Hu HH. Internal jugular vein reflux in patients with transient global amnesia: a meta-analysis of case-control studies. Acta Neurol Belg. 2012;112:237–44.

30. Bolwig TG. Transient global amnesia. Acta Neurol Scand. 1968;44:101–6.
31. Poser CM, Ziegler DK. Temporary amnesia as a manifestation of cerebrovascular insufficiency. Trans Am Neurol Assoc. 1960;85:221–3.
32. Whitty CWM, Lishman WA. Amnesia in cerebral disease. In: Whitty CWM, Zangwill OL, editors. Amnesia. London: Butterworths; 1966. p. 36–76.
33. Frederiks JAM. Transient global amnesia: an amnesic TIA. In: Markowitsch HJ, editor. Transient global amnesia and related disorders. Toronto: Hogrefe and Huber; 1990. p. 28–47.
34. Larner AJ. Transient global amnesia in the district general hospital. Int J Clin Pract. 2007;61:255–8.
35. Hodges JR. Transient amnesia. Clinical and neuropsychological aspects. London: WB Saunders; 1991.
36. Klötzsch C, Sliwka U, Berlit P, Noth J. An increased frequency of patent foramen ovale in patients with transient global amnesia. Analysis of 53 consecutive patients. Arch Neurol. 1996;53:504–8.
37. Caplan L, Chedru F, Lhermitte F, Mayman C. Transient global amnesia and migraine. Neurology. 1981;31:1167–70.
38. Toledo M, Pujadas F, Grivé E, Alvarez-Sabin J, Quintana M, Rovira A. Lack of evidence for arterial ischemia in transient global amnesia. Stroke. 2008;39:476–9.
39. Zola-Morgan S, Squire LR, Amaral DG. Human amnesia and the medial temporal region: enduring memory impairment following a bilateral lesion limited to field CA1 of the hippocampus. J Neurosci. 1986;6:2950–67.
40. Baracchini C, Farina F, Ballotta E, Meneghetti G, Manara R. No signs of intracranial arterial vasoconstriction in transient global amnesia. J Neuroimaging. 2015;25:92–6.
41. Lewis SL. Aetiology of transient global amnesia. Lancet. 1998;352:397–9.
42. Alblas CL, Beneder PR, Bulens C. Transient global amnesia: indications for a syndrome involving cerebral venous stasis [in Dutch]. Ned Tijdschr Geneeskd. 2006;150:1685–8.
43. Menendez-Gonzalez M, Rivera MM. Transient global amnesia: increasing evidence of a venous etiology. Arch Neurol. 2006;63:1334–6.
44. Baracchini C, Tonello S, Farina F, et al. Jugular veins in transient global amnesia: innocent bystanders. Stroke. 2012;43:2289–92.
45. Lochner P, Nedelmann M, Kaps M, Stolz E. Jugular valve incompetence in transient global amnesia. A problem revisited. J Neuroimaging. 2014;24:479–83.
46. Caplan LR. Transient global amnesia and jugular vein incompetence. Stroke. 2010;41:e568.
47. Bartsch T, Alfke K, Stingele R, et al. Selective affection of hippocampal CA-1 neurons in patients with transient global amnesia without long-term sequelae. Brain. 2006;129:2874–84.
48. Gomez-Choco M, Mariaca AF, Gaebel C, Valdueza JM. A controlled Valsalva maneuver causes neither diffusion-positive hippocampal lesions nor clinical symptoms after transient global amnesia. Eur Neurol. 2019;82:113–5.
49. Solheim O, Skeidsvoll T. Transient global amnesia may be caused by cerebral vein thrombosis. Med Hypotheses. 2005;65:1142–9.
50. Fisher CM. Transient global amnesia. Precipitating activities and other observations. Arch Neurol. 1982;39:605–8.
51. Crowell GF, Stump DA, Biller J, McHenry LC Jr, Toole JF. The transient global amnesia-migraine connection. Arch Neurol. 1984;41:75–9.
52. Santoro G, Casadei B, Venco A. The transient global amnesia-migraine connection. Case report. Funct Neurol. 1988;3:353–60.
53. Lane R, Davies P. Migraine. New York: Taylor & Francis; 2006.
54. Larner AJ. Late onset migraine with aura: how old is too old? J Headache Pain. 2007;8:251–2.
55. Larner AJ. Transient acute neurologic sequelae of sexual activity: headache and amnesia. J Sex Med. 2008;5:284–8.
56. Leão AAP. Spreading depression of activity in the cerebral cortex. J Neurophysiol. 1944;7:359–90.

57. Milner PM. Note on a possible correspondence between the scotomas of migraine and spreading depression of Leão. Electroencephalogr Clin Neurophysiol. 1958;10:705.
58. Lauritzen M. On the possible relation of spreading cortical depression to classical migraine. Cephalalgia. 1985;5(Suppl2):47–51.
59. Pearce JM. Is migraine explained by Leão's spreading depression? Lancet. 1985;2:763–6.
60. Olesen J, Jorgensen MB. Leao's spreading depression in the hippocampus explains transient global amnesia. A hypothesis. Acta Neurol Scand. 1986;73:219–20.
61. Larner AJ. Recurrent transient global amnesia: is there a link to familial history? Prog Neurol Psychiatry. 2017;21(4):17–9.
62. Segers-van Rijn J, de Bruijn SFTM. Transient global amnesia: a genetic disorder? Eur Neurol. 2010;63:186–7.
63. Arena JE, Rabinstein AA. In reply—familial transient global amnesia. Mayo Clin Proc. 2015;90:697.
64. Dupuis M, Vandeponseele M, Jacquerye P, et al. Familial transient global amnesia: report of 10 families. J Neurol Sci. 2017;381(Suppl):381.
65. Larner AJ. Recurrent TGA: link to family history? Prog Neurol Psychiatry. 2018;22(1):18.
66. Agosti C, Borroni B, Archetti S, Akkawi N, Padovani A. The brain-derived neurotrophic factor (BDNF) Val66Met polymorphism is not significantly correlated to transient global amnesia: preliminary results of an on-going study in Brescia Province. Italy Neurosci Lett. 2008;443:228–31.
67. Schmitz B, Tettenborn B, Schomer DL, editors. The paroxysmal disorders. Cambridge: Cambridge University Press; 2010.
68. Park KM, Lee BI, Kim SE. Is transient global amnesia a network disease? Eur Neurol. 2018;80:345–54.
69. Kanzer M. Amnesia. A statistical study. Am J Psychiatry. 1939;96:711–6.
70. Kennedy A, Neville J. Sudden loss of memory. BMJ. 1957;2:428–33.
71. Merriam AE. Emotional arousal-induced transient global amnesia. Case report, differentiation from hysterical amnesia, and an etiologic hypothesis. Neuropsychiatry Neuropsychol Behav Neurol. 1988;1:73–8.
72. Larner AJ. Transient global amnesia. From patient encounter to clinical neuroscience. London: Springer; 2017.
73. Cho HJ, Sung YH, Lee SH, Chung JY, Kang JM, Yi JW. Isoflurane induces transient anterograde amnesia through suppression of brain-derived neurotrophic factor in hippocampus. J Korean Neurosurg Soc. 2013;53:139–44.
74. Kesner RP, Dixon DA, Pickett D, Berman RF. Experimental animal model of transient global amnesia: role of the hippocampus. Neuropsychologia. 1975;13:465–80.
75. Morgan RE, Burch-Vernon AS, Riccio DC. Experimental induction of retrograde and anterograde amnesia concurrently: an animal model. Psychobiology. 1993;21:221–7.
76. Castellani JW, Young AJ, Sawka MN, Backus VL, Canete JJ. Amnesia during cold water immersion: a case report. Wilderness Environ Med. 1998;9:153–5.
77. Hodges JR, Warlow CP. Syndromes of transient amnesia: towards a classification. A study of 153 cases. J Neurol Neurosurg Psychiatry. 1990;53:834–43.
78. Baezner H, Blahak C, Capelle HH, Schrader C, Lutjens G, Krauss JK. Transient global amnesia associated with accidental high-frequency stimulation of the right hippocampus in deep brain stimulation for segmental dystonia. Stereotact Funct Neurosurg. 2013;91:335–7.
79. Glannon W. The neuroethics of memory. From total recall to oblivion. Cambridge: Cambridge University Press; 2019.
80. Meeter M, Murre JMJ. TraceLink: a model of consolidation and amnesia. Cogn Neuropsychol. 2005;22:559–87.
81. Marr D. Simple memory: a theory for archicortex. Philos Trans R Soc Lond Ser B Biol Sci. 1971;262:23–81.
82. Murre JMJ, Chessa AG, Meeter M. A mathematical model of forgetting and amnesia. Front Psychol. 2013;4:76.

83. Kritchevsky M, Squire LR. Transient global amnesia: evidence for extensive, temporally graded retrograde amnesia. Neurology. 1989;39:213–9.
84. Broadbent SR, Hammersley JM. Percolation processes. I. Crystals and mazes. Math Proc Camb Philos Soc. 1957;53:629–41.
85. George D, Hawkins J. Towards a mathematical theory of cortical micro-circuits. PLoS Comput Biol. 2009;5:e1000532.
86. Swanson N, Swanson LW. (transl.). Histology of the nervous system of man and vertebrates by S Ramón y Cajal, vol. 2nd. New York: Oxford University Press; [1911.] 1995. p. 626–57.
87. Andersen P, Bliss TVP, Skrede KK. Lamellar organization of hippocampal excitatory pathways. Exp Brain Res. 1971;13:222–38.
88. Lorente de Nó R. Studies on the structure of the cerebral cortex. II. Continuation of the study of the ammonic system. J Psychol Neurol. 1934;46:113–77.
89. Schaffer K. Beitrag zur Histologie der Ammonshornformation. Arch Mikrosk Anat. 1892;39:611–32.
90. van Haeften T, Baks-te-Bulte L, Goede PH, Wouterlood FG, Witter MP. Morphological and numerical analysis of synaptic interactions between neurons in deep and superficial layers of the entorhinal cortex of the rat. Hippocampus. 2003;13:943–52.
91. Hsu D. The dentate gyrus as a filter or gate: a look back and a look ahead. Prog Brain Res. 2007;163:601–13.
92. Rebola N, Carta M, Mulle C. Operation and plasticity of hippocampal CA3 circuits: implications for memory encoding. Nat Rev Neurosci. 2017;18:209–21.
93. Cobb M. The idea of the brain. A history. London: Profile Books; 2020.
94. Heims SJ. Constructing a social science for postwar America. The cybernetics group, 1946–1953. Cambridge: MIT Press; 1991.
95. Hebb DO. The organization of behavior: a neuropsychological theory. New York: Wiley; 1949.
96. Brindley GS. Nerve net models of plausible size that perform many simple learning tasks. Proc R Soc Lond B Biol Sci. 1969;174:173–91.
97. Barlow H, Levick WR. The mechanism of directionally selective units in rabbit's retina. J Physiol. 1965;178:477–504.
98. Bennett MR, Gibson WG, Robinson J. Dynamics of the CA3 pyramidal neuron autoassociative memory network in the hippocampus. Philos Trans R Soc Lond Ser B Biol Sci. 1994;343:167–87.
99. Bennett MR, Hacker PMS. Philosophical foundations of neuroscience. Oxford: Blackwell; 2003.
100. Bennett MR, Hacker PMS. History of cognitive neuroscience. Chichester: Wiley-Blackwell; 2008. 2013.
101. Kesner RP, Rolls ET. A computational theory of hippocampal function, and tests of the theory: new developments. Neurosci Biobehav Rev. 2015;48:92–147.
102. Knierim JJ, Neunuebel JP. Tracking the flow of hippocampal computation: pattern separation, pattern completion, and attractor dynamics. Neurobiol Learn Mem. 2016;129:38–49.
103. Rolls ET. Cerebral cortex. Principles of operation. Oxford: Oxford University Press; 2016.
104. Rolls ET. Attractor network dynamics, transmitters, and memory and cognitive changes in aging. In: Heilman KM, Nadeau SE, editors. Cognitive changes and the aging brain. Cambridge: Cambridge University Press; 2019. p. 203–25.
105. Larner AJ. Transient global amnesia: model, mechanism, hypothesis. Cortex. 2022;149:137–47.
106. Hanert A, Pedersen A, Bartsch T. Transient hippocampal CA1 lesions in humans impair pattern separation performance. Hippocampus. 2019;29:736–47.
107. Hodges JR. Unraveling the enigma of transient global amnesia. Ann Neurol. 1998;43:151–3.
108. Strupp M, Brüning R, Wu RH, Deimling M, Reiser M, Brandt T. Diffusion-weighted MRI in transient global amnesia: elevated signal intensity in the left mesial temporal lobe in 7 out of 10 patients. Ann Neurol. 1998;43:164–70.
109. Ding X, Peng D. Transient global amnesia: an electrophysiological disorder based on cortical spreading depression-transient global amnesia model. Front Hum Neurosci. 2020;14:602496.

110. Ayata C, Lauritzen M. Spreading depression, spreading depolarizations, and the cerebral vasculature. Physiol Rev. 2015;95:953–93.
111. Cozzolino O, Marchese M, Trovato F, et al. Understanding spreading depression from headache to sudden unexpected death. Front Neurol. 2018;9:19.
112. Hartings JA, Shuttleworth CW, Kirov SA, et al. The continuum of spreading depolarizations in acute cortical lesion development: examining Leão's legacy. J Cereb Blood Flow Metab. 2017;37:1571–94.
113. Hübers A, Thoma K, Schocke M, et al. Acute DWI reductions in patients after single epileptic seizures – more common than assumed. Front Neurol. 2018;9:550.
114. Larner AJ. Migralepsy explained … perhaps½. Adv Clin Neurosci Rehabil. 2021;20(4):32–3.
115. Ung KYC, Larner AJ. Transient amnesia: epileptic or global? A differential diagnosis with significant implications for management. Q J Med. 2014;107:915–7.
116. Dreier JP, Woitzik J, Fabricius M, et al. Delayed ischaemic neurological deficits after subarachnoid haemorrhage are associated with clusters of spreading depolarizations. Brain. 2006;129:3224–37.
117. Paech D, Kuder TA, Roßmanith C, et al. What remains after transient global amnesia (TGA)? An ultra-high field 7T magnetic resonance imaging study of the hippocampus. Eur J Neurol. 2020;27:406–9.
118. Barry DN, Tierney TM, Holmes N, et al. Imaging the human hippocampus with optically-pumped magnetoencephalography. NeuroImage. 2019;203:116192.
119. Li Y, Wang T, Zhang T, et al. Fast high-resolution metabolic imaging of acute stroke with 3D magnetic resonance spectroscopy. Brain. 2020;143:3225–33.
120. Bastany ZJR, Askari S, Dumont GA, Kellinghaus C, Kazemi A, Gorji A. Association of cortical spreading depression and seizures with medically intractable epilepsy. Clin Neurophysiol. 2020;131:2861–74.
121. Hertelendy P, Varga DP, Menyhart A, Bari F, Farkas E. Susceptibility of the cerebral cortex to spreading depolarization in neurological disease states: the impact of aging. Neurochem Int. 2019;127:125–36.
122. Bartsch T, Döhring J, Reuter S, et al. Selective neuronal vulnerability of human hippocampal CA1 neurons: lesion evolution, temporal course, and pattern of hippocampal damage in diffusion-weighted MR imaging. J Cereb Blood Flow Metab. 2015;35:1836–45.
123. Schmidt-Kastner R, Freund TF. Selective vulnerability of the hippocampus in brain ischemia. Neuroscience. 1991;40:599–636.
124. Spielmeyer W. Zur Pathogenese örtlich elektiver Gehirnveränderungen. Z Ges Neurol Psychiatr. 1925;99:756–76.
125. Medvedeva YV, Ji SG, Yin HZ, Weiss JH. Differential vulnerability of CA1 versus CA3 neurons after ischemia: possible relationship to sources of Zn^{2+} accumulation and its entry into and prolonged effects on mitochondria. J Neurosci. 2017;37:726–37.
126. Förster A, Griebe M, Gass A, Kern R, Hennerici MG, Szabo K. Diffusion-weighted imaging for the differential diagnosis of disorders affecting the hippocampus. Cerebrovasc Dis. 2012;33:104–15.

Index

Printed in the United States
by Baker & Taylor Publisher Services